Diabetes and Endocrine Disorders in Primary Care

RCGP Curriculum for
General Practice Series

Diabetes and Endocrine Disorders in Primary Care

Roger Gadsby MBE

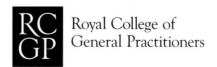

Royal College of
General Practitioners

The Royal College of General Practitioners was founded in 1952 with this object:

'To encourage, foster and maintain the highest possible standards in general practice and for that purpose to take or join with others in taking steps consistent with the charitable nature of that object which may assist towards the same.'

Among its responsibilities under its Royal Charter the College is entitled to:

'Diffuse information on all matters affecting general practice and issue such publications as may assist the object of the College.'

British Library Cataloguing-in-Publication Data
A catalogue record for this book is available from the British Library

Disclaimer

This publication is intended for the use of medical practitioners in the UK and not for patients. The authors, editors and publisher have taken care to ensure that the information contained in this book is correct to the best of their knowledge, at the time of publication. Whilst efforts have been made to ensure the accuracy of the information presented, particularly that related to the prescription of drugs, the authors, editors and publisher cannot accept liability for information that is subsequently shown to be wrong. Readers are advised to check that the information, especially that related to drug usage, complies with information contained in the *British National Formulary*, or equivalent, or manufacturers' datasheets, and that it complies with the latest legislation and standards of practice.

Designed and typeset at the Typographic Design Unit
Printed by Hobbs the Printers Ltd
Indexed by Carol Ball

ISBN: 978-0-85084-325-5

Contents

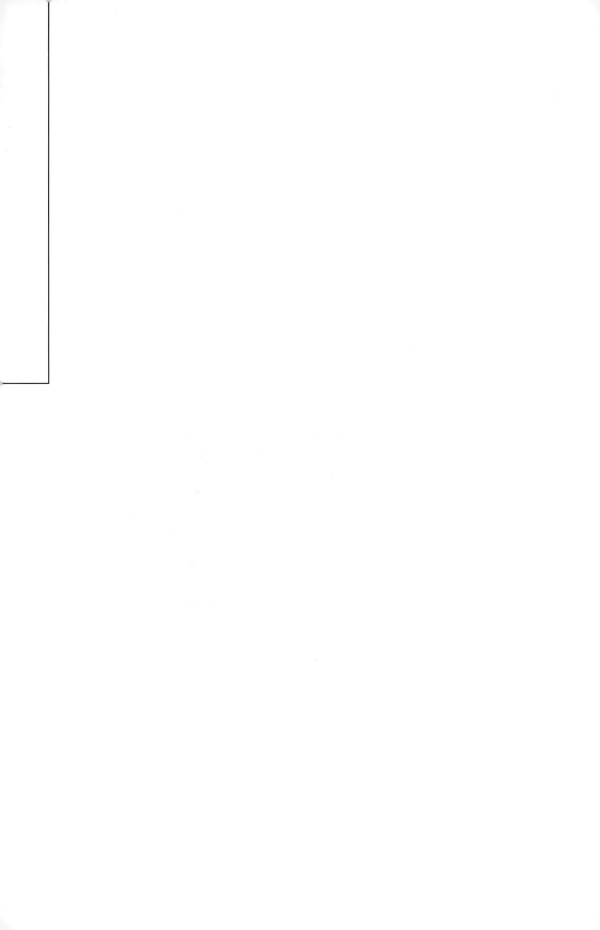

Preface

This book has been written as part of the RCGP Curriculum in General Practice Series. It expands on curriculum statement 15.6, *Metabolic Problems*, produced for the nMRCGP assessment.

General practitioners in the UK encounter a variety of metabolic problems. These range from the very common, such as obesity and diabetes, to the very rare, such as Addison's and Cushing's disease.

The 'average' practice of 10,000 patients, according to the published levels of prevalence, would have the following numbers of patients:

▷ 400 with diabetes
▷ 250 with hypothyroidism
▷ 100 with hyperthyroidism
▷ 4.5 with hypopituitism
▷ 1.2 with Addison's
▷ 0.05 with primary Cushing's disease.

This book contains practical information about both the rare and common metabolic problems, with an emphasis on the common condition of diabetes. Case scenarios embed the teaching and each chapter summary relates the contents of the chapter to the six domains of core or essential competences of being a GP

I am very grateful to my colleague Dr Vinod Patel, Consultant Physician at the George Eliot Hospital, Nuneaton, and Reader in Medical Education at the Warwick Medical School for reviewing the endocrine chapters and for writing the Foreword.

I am also indebted to Dr Rodger Charlton for all his help and editorial advice in writing this book.

Roger Gadsby
University of Warwick
July 2009

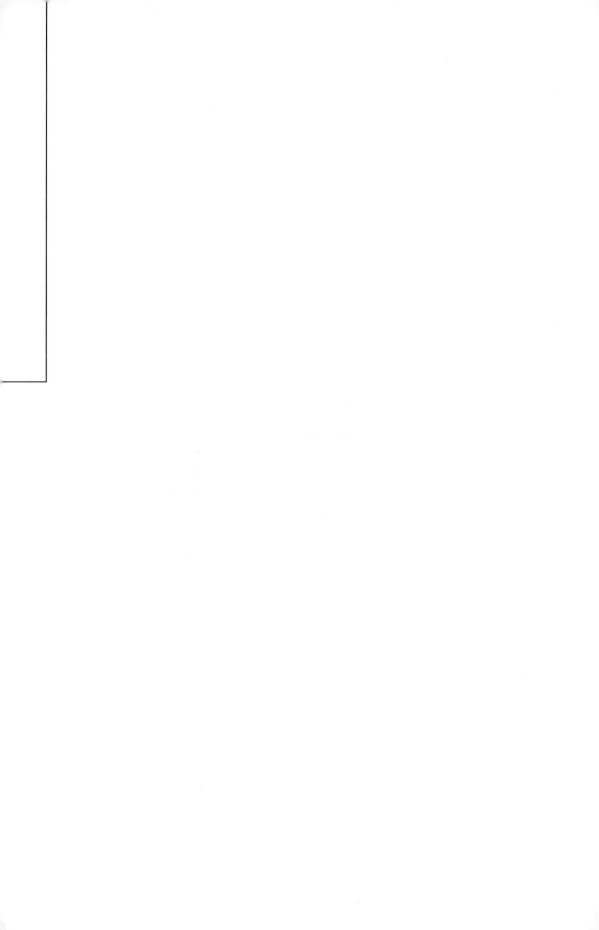

Foreword

There is no doubt in my mind that this book will become one of the most used resources for the management of patients with diabetes and endocrine disorders in clinical care. Although presented predominantly for a primary care audience, it will be of considerable value to clinicians in secondary care as well. The book covers the broad sweep of all the main clinical areas in diabetes and endocrinology, including: obesity; diagnosis of diabetes; macrovascular and microvascular complications; glycaemic control and the newer agents; ethnic and psycho-social aspects of care; and structure of care.

Roger Gadsby usually describes himself as a jobbing GP. This we cannot take away from him, as he has been an extremely busy clinician running an excellent service in diabetes care for at least 25 years. Indeed, his GP diabetes clinic was one of the first of its kind in the UK. His clinical knowledge contributes greatly to the quality of the factual material, and his clinical experience is disseminated to the reader on every page.

Roger has been involved in the writing of several national guidelines, including the NICE guideline for Type 2 diabetes in 2008 and the subsequent amendments in May 2009. He is also an academic attached to Warwick Medical School, University of Warwick. His academic rigour as associate professor thus comes across in the presentations of the evidence base for the management decisions and concise summaries of key randomised clinical trials, such as UKPDS, which have influenced clinical care. The clinical vignettes discussed are realistic and closely mirror common clinical encounters in general practice. The real innovation in this particular book is to deal with thyroid and some rarer endocrine disorders, including pituitary disease. Roger thereby addresses a clinical education need that is rarely tackled. This will be a particularly useful section.

Personally, this book fits in with a philosophy of health care that we teach to summarise the many diverse views on how to conduct effective health care. Throughout, healthcare delivery is presented as needing to be patient centred, outcome based, evidence based, team delivered, integrated (holistic) and cost-effective but clinically governed. This book will inspire clinicians to deliver this POETIC vision. Clinical care will be enhanced and the lives of patients with diabetes improved.

Vinod Patel
University of Warwick
July 2009

Abbreviations

A : C ratio	albumin : creatinine ratio
ACE	angiotensin-converting enzyme
ACTH	adrenocorticotrophic hormone
ADH	antidiuretic hormone
APA	aldosterone-producing adenoma
ARB	angiotensin receptor blocker
AT2s	angiotensin 2 antagonists
b.d.	twice a day
BMI	body mass index
CARDS	Collaborative Atorvastatin Diabetes Study
CB1	central cannabinoid 1
cGMP	cyclic guanosine monophosphate
CHD	coronary heart disease
CIDC	Certificate in Diabetes Care
CKD	chronic kidney disease
CVD	cardiovascular disease
DAFNE	dose adjustment for normal eating
DCCT	Diabetes Control and Complications Trial
DKA	diabetic ketoacidosis
DPP-4	dipeptidyl peptidase-4
DSN	diabetes specialist nurse
DVLA	Driver and Vehicle Licensing Agency
ED	erectile dysfunction
eGFR	estimated glomerular filtration rate
ESR	erythrocyte sedimentation rate
FSH	follicle-stimulating hormone
GDM	Gestational Diabetes Mellitus
GH	growth hormone
GI	gastrointestinal
GIP	glucose-dependent insulinotropic polypeptide
GLP-1	glucagon-like peptide-1
GPwSI	GP with a Special Interest
HCA	healthcare assistant
HDL	high-density lipoprotein
HONK	hyperosmolar non-ketotic state
HPS	Heart Protection Study
HSS	hyperosmolar hyperglycaemic state

IDF	International Diabetes Federation
IFG	impaired fasting glucose
IGT	impaired glucose tolerance
IM	intramuscular
ITU	Intensive Treatment Unit
IV	intravenous
LES	locally enhanced services
LH	luteinising hormone
LVD	left ventricular dysfunction
MSH	melanocyte-stimulating hormone
NPH	neutral protamine Hagedorn
OGTT	oral glucose tolerance test
PAC	plasma aldosterone concentration
PBC	Practice-Based Commissioning
PCDS	Primary Care Diabetes Society
PCOS	polycystic ovary syndrome
PDE	phosphodiesterase type 5
PRA	plasma rennin activity
QoF	Quality and Outcomes Framework
SAH	subarachnoid haemorrhage
SC	subcutaneous
SMBG	self-monitoring of blood glucose
SNRI	serotonin and norepinephrine reuptake inhibitor
t.d.s.	three times a day
TPO	thyroid peroxidase
TSH	thyroid-stimulating hormone
UKADS	United Kingdom Asian Diabetes Study
UKPDS	United Kingdom Prospective Diabetes Study
UTI	urinary tract infection

Obesity

Scenario

John, a 45-year-old patient, comes to see you because he is desperate to lose weight. He realises he has been significantly overweight for the past 15 years and is now having difficulty breathing when he tries to walk upstairs or hurry to catch a bus. He thinks his weight has gone up in the past 12 months as his marriage has broken up and he says he has been 'comfort eating'. He has not dared to weigh himself for the last few months but thinks he must weigh around 20 st. He is a non-smoker and has had no significant past medical history. He is on no medications.

On clinical examination he weighs 21 st., which gives him a body mass index (BMI) of 38 kg/m². His blood pressure is 150/90 but there are no other abnormal signs.

▶ *What actions would you take?*

Background

In many countries of the world, including the UK, there is a rising tide of obesity. The World Health Organization (WHO) has described obesity as one of the most blatantly visible, yet most neglected, public health problems threatening both developed and developing countries.[1]

There is a very close correlation between increasing weight and the incidence of diabetes, hypertension, dyslipidaemia and cardiovascular disease, which contributes to the estimated cost of obesity to the NHS in the UK of over £500 million and to the wider economy of £2 billion.[2]

Definitions of obesity

In Caucasian populations a BMI at or above 30 is considered as obese, and a BMI between 25 and 29.9 is considered as overweight. Morbid obesity is defined as a BMI at or above 40.[3]

In Indo-Asian populations there is a move to lower thresholds of BMI with some suggesting that 23–26.9 be considered as overweight and 27 and above be considered obese. This is because in these populations there seems to be a higher prevalence of obesity-related complications at lower levels of BMI.[4]

Epidemiology of obesity in the UK

The rates of obesity are rapidly rising in the UK. They almost tripled between 1980 and 1998 from 8 per cent of women and 6 per cent of men to 21 and 17 per cent respectively.[2] In 2005 22 per cent of English men and 24 per cent of English women were classified as obese, as were 18 per cent of boys and girls aged 2–15 years.

The recently published report on obesities in the UK entitled *Tackling Obesities*[5] predicted that, by 2050, 60 per cent of men and 50 per cent of women could be clinically obese.

Obesity and the Quality and Outcomes Framework

In the 2006/7 Quality and Outcomes Framework (QoF) round of the GP contract there was one clinical indicator for obesity that was worth 8 points. It was that the practice could produce a register of patients aged 16 and over with a BMI greater or equal to 30 in the previous 12 months. The 8372 practices in the UK achieved 100 per cent of the total points available for this clinical indicator and the recorded prevalence of obesity was 7.4 per cent across all age ranges.[6]

Causes of obesity

Obesity occurs where there is an imbalance between calorie intake and energy exertion through exercise. On a population level we are eating more, and find ourselves bombarded with advertising that encourages us to eat very energy-dense 'junk foods'. We also live in an environment that often discourages exercise through our dependence on car travel, use of labour-saving devices and limited access to affordable exercise facilities.

Treatment of obesity

At population level

At the population level tackling obesity requires significant political will to discourage overeating and promote exercise. Many initiatives are being taken by the government in the UK, including ones to reduce the advertising of junk foods, to encourage healthy eating, and to promote physical activity.

At individual level

At the individual level primary care spends a lot of time treating and managing patients when they develop conditions associated with obesity, such as diabetes, hypertension and cardiovascular disease (CVD). We also see many obese patients before they have developed these associated conditions.

There is scant evidence that short primary care interventions can effectively help patients with obesity to lose weight and to keep that weight from returning.[4]

There is a good evidence base in patients with impaired glucose tolerance that intensive lifestyle change (weight loss and increased exercise) can reduce the progression to frank diabetes from both the Diabetes Prevention Programme[7] and a study conducted in Finland.[8] However, both studies had intensive input from trained professionals to deliver and support lifestyle change. Resources like this are just not available in every primary care service in the UK.

The 2006 NICE obesity guideline[3] recommends that at an initial consultation with someone who is obese the healthcare professional should raise the issue of weight and then assess lifestyle, co-morbidities and willingness to change. If there is no willingness to change, some guidelines suggest just giving brief written information such as the leaflet *Why Weight Matters.*[9]

If there is willingness to change, the NICE guideline recommends that a multicomponent intervention is offered that is designed to increase physical activity, improve eating behaviour and encourage healthy eating. The recommendation for physical activity is to do at least 30 minutes of at least moderate-intensity physical activity (such as brisk walking) on five or more days a week. It also states that patients who have lost weight may need to do 60–90 minutes to avoid regaining weight.

The detailed recommendations for dietary change are listed in the guideline and basically involve individualised healthy eating advice with the aim of losing a maximum of 0.5–1 kg weekly. The guideline suggests that commercial, community and/or self-help management programmes can be helpful if these meet best-practice standards. Follow-up to monitor weight and to provide support and care is recommended.

3

Drug therapy for obesity

Drug therapy for weight loss should be considered only after dietary, exercise and behavioural approaches have been started and evaluated. It should be considered for patients who have not reached their target weight loss or have reached a plateau on dietary, exercise and behavioural changes alone.

The NICE 2006 guideline[3] provides advice on the use of two agents: orlistat and sibutramine. It advises that one or other be prescribed only as part of an overall plan for managing obesity in adults who have a BMI of 28 or more with associated risk factors (BMI of 27 or more for sibutramine) or a BMI of 30 or more without risk factors.

It advises that treatment only be continued for longer than 3 months if the person has lost at least 5 per cent of his or her initial body weight. However, the guideline states that less strict goals may be appropriate in patients with Type 2 diabetes.

Orlistat treatment can be continued for longer than 12 months. Orlistat is a lipase inhibitor that acts in the gastrointestinal (GI) tract to inhibit absorption of fats. Its main side effect is fatty diarrhoea, which occurs mainly when patients cheat on the diet and eat fatty foods.

Sibutramine is a centrally acting serotonin and norepinephrine reuptake inhibitor (SNRI) that acts as an appetite suppressant. Sibutramine treatment may be associated with adverse effects of tachycardia and raised blood pressure, and patients taking it must be regularly monitored for these events. It is contraindicated in patients with cardiovascular disease and uncontrolled hypertension. Sibutramine treatment is not recommended beyond the licence duration of 12 months.

Surgical treatment for obesity

The usual surgical procedure is gastric banding. NICE recommends that surgery be considered as a first-line option for adults with a BMI of more than 50 kg/m² in whom surgical intervention is considered appropriate.[3] Use of orlistat and sibutramine before surgery should be considered if the waiting time is long.

It also recommends that surgery be considered for patients with severe obesity if:

1 ▷ they have a BMI of 40 kg/m² or more, or between 35–40 and other significant disease (for example Type 2 diabetes or hypertension)
2 ▷ all appropriate non-surgical measures have failed to achieve or maintain adequate clinically beneficial weight loss for at least 6 months

3 ▷ they are receiving or will receive intensive specialist management
4 ▷ they are generally fit for anaesthesia and surgery
5 ▷ they commit to the need for long-term follow-up.

The guideline recommends that the surgery be performed only by a surgeon with the appropriate training and skills who is part of a multidisciplinary team.

Treating obesity in individuals to prevent diabetes

Reducing weight can delay or prevent diabetes in groups at risk of developing Type 2 diabetes [7,8] and in obese people generally. [5]

A Finnish study among 522 middle-aged, overweight subjects with impaired glucose tolerance (IGT), who are at significantly increased risk for Type 2 diabetes, clearly showed that an active programme of increased physical activity and dietary change can prevent the onset of the disease. [8] When compared with routine care, individualised counselling for lifestyle changes resulted in an increased level of physical activity and a significant loss of weight: mean loss of 3.5 ± 5.5 kg after 2 years. This active treatment conferred a 58 per cent reduction in the risk for developing diabetes; the cumulative incidence of diabetes after 4 years being 11 per cent compared with 23 per cent in the control group receiving routine care.

Further evidence on the effectiveness of nutrition and exercise therapy in preventing diabetes developing in people with IGT, who are at very significant risk of developing diabetes, comes from the Heart Protection study from the USA. [7] In this study several thousand people with IGT were divided into groups. One group received a diet and exercise programme that was aimed at achieving a weight reduction of around 7 per cent, and taking part in moderate physical activity, for example brisk walking for 150 minutes per week. People in this active arm of the study had regular one-to-one sessions with their case manager in the first 24 weeks, and then monthly sessions for the remaining period of the study. Fifty per cent of people achieved the weight reduction target at 24 weeks and 74 per cent achieved the exercise target.

When compared with the control group who received 'general advice' those in the lifestyle and exercise group reduced their risk of developing diabetes by 58 per cent, exactly the same risk reduction as in the Finnish study.

Another approach to reducing the incidence of diabetes that has been tested in a randomised controlled trial has been the use, in combination with lifestyle change, of the lipase inhibitor orlistat, which acts locally in the gut to reduce absorption of ingested fat. In the XENDOS study, carried out in 22 centres in

Sweden, 3304 obese individuals, 21 per cent of whom had IGT, were given life-style advice and either placebo or orlistat 120 mg t.d.s., and were followed for 4 years. Those receiving orlistat lost on average 6.9 kg in weight against 4.1 kg on placebo. The cumulative incidence of Type 2 diabetes was 9 per cent in the lifestyle plus placebo group and 6.2 per cent in the lifestyle plus orlistat group, a risk reduction of 37 per cent. This study shows that in an obese population, in which 21 per cent had IGT, orlistat together with lifestyle change over 4 years resulted in a greater weight loss and a significantly reduced incidence of Type 2 diabetes as compared with intensive lifestyle changes alone. Orlistat was well tolerated in the study.[10]

Scenario revisited

John accepts your advice to increase his amount of physical activity and to diet to lose weight. He agrees to see the practice nurse every 2 weeks for weight monitoring and to see you again in 8 weeks.

At 8 weeks John has lost 1 st. in weight, feels better in himself and says he feels less breathless. His blood pressure is now 140/80. He agrees to continue to see the practice nurse monthly for weighing.

He comes to see you again 6 months later. He weighs 17 st. and his blood pressure is 130/80. He says how well he feels and how his life is now so much more settled. He is planning to get married to the lovely lady he met just over 6 months ago!

Metabolic syndrome

The association of visceral adiposity, dyslipidaemia, hypertension and hyper-glycaemia has been known about for over 80 years but received scant attention till 1988 when Reaven described the constellation as Syndrome X. Various names were subsequently proposed but metabolic syndrome seems to be the one that is in most widespread use. Reaven thought that insulin resistance was the cause but this remains uncertain.[11] There have been several defini-tions put forward but in 2005 a consensus group from the International Dia-betes Federation (IDF) proposed a definition that requires a person to have:

▷ central obesity defined by a series of ethnically specific waist
  circumference measures; in Europids [Caucasians] they are 94 cm
  or more for men and 80 cm or more for women

plus any two of:

▷ raised triglycerides above 1.7 mmol/l or treatment for this lipid abnormality
▷ reduced HDL cholesterol, below 1.03 mmol/l for men or 1.29 mmol/l for women, or treatment for this lipid abnormality
▷ raised blood pressure at or above 130/85 or treatment for previously diagnosed hypertension
▷ raised fasting glucose at or above 5.6 mmol/l or previously diagnosed Type 2 diabetes.

The authors of the definition state that their aim is to help in the identification of a group of people at high risk of CVD and diabetes.

They state that the treatment of the metabolic syndrome should be focused on lifestyle change and on individual components of the syndrome if this fails.[11]

There is still much debate about whether the risk associated with the condition is greater than the sum of the individual parts or whether the underlying problem is obesity and all the other components are 'downstream' of this.

The IDF definition of metabolic syndrome does require the measurement of waist circumference rather than just using BMI as a measure of obesity. Measurement of waist circumference is as yet not part of the QoF of the new GP contract and is not routinely performed in primary care. In my opinion it is likely to become a QoF requirement in the near future.

Treatment of the metabolic syndrome should be directed at weight reduction through diet and exercise, and the treatment of its individual components, e.g. hypertension and dyslipidaemia. These are discussed in later chapters.

Polycystic ovary syndrome

In 1935 Stein and Leventhal first described the polycystic ovary as a frequent cause of irregular ovulation in women seeking treatment for subfertility. The use of abdominal ultrasound has now shown that many women have the ultrasound characteristics of polycystic ovaries with or without the biochemical or clinical features of polycystic ovary syndrome (PCOS). The association between increased insulin resistance and PCOS is a consistent finding in all ethnic groups. Obesity is also a common finding in many women with PCOS.[12]

Epidemiology of PCOS

It is the most common endocrine disorder, affecting about 1 in 15 women worldwide.[13]

Causes of PCOS

It is a heterogeneous familial condition of uncertain aetiology. Insulin resistance of the ovary has been postulated as the underlying pathophysiological abnormality, putting PCOS as possibly part of the metabolic syndrome.

Features of PCOS

The major endocrine problem is excessive androgen secretion or activity that results in menstrual cycle disturbances, subfertility, obesity, hirsutism and acne.

There is a significantly increased risk of developing Type 2 diabetes, and associations with dyslipidaemia and hypertension, suggesting that women with PCOS may be more likely to develop cardiovascular disease later in life.

People with PCOS often first present with symptoms of subfertility, period problems or hirsutism, or a combination of these.

Management of PCOS

Referral to a gynaecological endocrinologist or other specialist with an interest in PCOS is helpful for diagnosis and management. Lifestyle advice should be given to encourage increased physical activity and weight loss, which are the first-line treatments in women with PCOS, particularly in those who are overweight. This often results in the improvement of symptoms and endocrine profile. Specific treatments may need to be directed at specific symptoms. Menstrual cycle regulation may be achieved using the combined oral contraceptive pill. Treatment with metformin, which reduces insulin resistance, has been used off licence in PCOS and has been found to restore periods, ovulation and fertility in some. Clomifene has also been used in some women with PCOS to induce ovulation. The surgical techniques of laparoscopic ovarian diathermy or drilling of the ovary have been used in some women.

Summary

In relation to the six domains of core or essential competences of being a GP:

1 Primary care management

▷ Recognition of obesity and metabolic syndrome as a public health and individual patient problem.
▷ Treatment with lifestyle, diet and exercise. Appropriate use of oral anti-obesity drugs.
▷ Recognition of PCOS and referral where indicated to an appropriate specialist.

2 Person-centred care

▷ Negotiation of appropriate lifestyle, diet and exercise interventions and targets for obese individuals.

3 Specific problem-solving skills

▷ Diagnosing PCOS.
▷ Recognising metabolic syndrome.

4 A comprehensive approach

▷ Diagnosing and managing the co-morbidities of hypertension, dyslipidaemia, renal impairment and increased coronary heart disease (CHD) risk in people with obesity and metabolic syndrome.

5 Community orientation

▷ Understanding the need for local interventions (e.g. organised walks, exercise on prescription schemes) to improve fitness and reduce obesity.

6 A holistic approach

▷ Exploring the implications of obesity and metabolic syndrome for the individual at work, at home and at leisure.

References

1 • World Health Organization. *Obesity: preventing and managing the global epidemic* (WHO technical report series no. 894) Geneva: WHO, 2000.

2 • National Audit Office. *Tackling Obesity in England: report by the Comptroller and Auditor General* London: The Stationery Office, 2001.

3 • National Institute for Health and Clinical Excellence. *Clinical Guideline 43, Obesity: guidance on the prevention, identification, assessment and management of overweight and obesity in adults and children* London: NICE, 2006, www.nice.org.uk/nicemedia/pdf/CG43NICEGuideline.pdf [accessed July 2009].

4 • Jarvis S. Obesity and the overworked GP *British Journal of General Practice* 2006; **56(530)**: 654–5.

5 • Foresight. *Tackling Obesities: future choices* London: Government Office for Science, 2007, www.foresight.gov.uk/OurWork/ActiveProjects/Obesity/KeyInfo/Index.asp [accessed July 2009].

6 • www.ic.nhs.uk/statistics-and-data-collections/audits-and-performance/the-quality-and-outcomes-framework [accessed July 2009].

7 • Diabetes Prevention Programme Research Group. Prevention of type 2 diabetes by changes in lifestyle among subjects with impaired glucose tolerance *New England Journal of Medicine* 2002; **346**: 393–403.

8 • Tuomilehto J, Lindstrom M S, Eriksson J G, *et al*. Prevention of type 2 diabetes mellitus by changes in lifestyle among subjects with impaired glucose tolerance *New England Journal of Medicine* 2001; **344**: 1343–9.

9 • Department of Health. *Why Weight Matters* London: Central Office of Information, 2006.

10 • Torgerson J S, Hauptman J, Boldrin M, *et al*. XENical in the prevention of Diabetes in Obese Subjects (XENDOS) study *Diabetes Care* 2004; **27**: 155–61.

11 • Alberti G M M, Zimmet P, Shaw J for the IDF Consensus Group. The metabolic syndrome: a new worldwide definition *Lancet* 2005; **366**: 1059–61.

12 • Vignesh J P, Mohan V. Polycystic ovary syndrome: a component of metabolic syndrome? *Journal of Postgraduate Medicine* 2007; **53**: 128–34.

13 • Norman R J, Dewally D, Legro R S, *et al*. Polycystic ovary syndrome *Lancet* 2007; **370**: 685–97.

Definitions and diagnosis of diabetes mellitus

2

Epidemiology and management

Scenario 1

Margaret, a 65-year-old woman, has had hypertension for 9 years. She is a retired bus driver. As part of her annual hypertension review she has a fasting glucose estimation included in her annual bloods. It comes back as 6.4 mmol/l. In previous years it has always been below 6. Margaret says she has put on a stone in weight in the past year. She weighs 15 st., giving her a BMI of 32. Her blood pressure is well controlled on ramipril 10 mg daily and bendroflumethiazide 2.5 mg daily. She takes simvastatin 40 mg daily for primary coronary heart disease (CHD) prevention and her total cholesterol is 4.4 mmol/l.

She feels well and is asymptomatic.

▶ *How would you further investigate and manage her blood glucose?*

Classification of diabetes

The World Health Organization (WHO) classifies diabetes into: [1]

▷ Type 1 diabetes, characterised by pancreatic beta cell destruction
▷ Type 2 diabetes
▷ other specific types – e.g. genetic, or associated with pancreatitis
▷ gestational – diabetes or impaired glucose tolerance (IGT) occurring in pregnancy.

Diagnosis of diabetes

The new WHO criteria for diagnosing diabetes were adopted in the UK on 1 June 2000.[2] These outline the criteria for diagnosing diabetes on fasting or random blood glucose measurements. The diagnostic criteria are the same for both Type 1 and Type 2 diabetes.

On fasting blood results

Diabetes is diagnosed as a fasting plasma glucose of 7 mmol/l and above (see Figure 2.1).

Figure 2.1 ○ *Fasting plasma glucose*

Diabetes diagnosed	**If asymptomatic repeat to confirm**
7.0 mmol/l	
Impaired fasting glucose	**Proceed to oral glucose tolerance test**
6.0 mmol/l	
Normal	**Repeat if screening protocol says so. In USA it is repeated every 3 years**

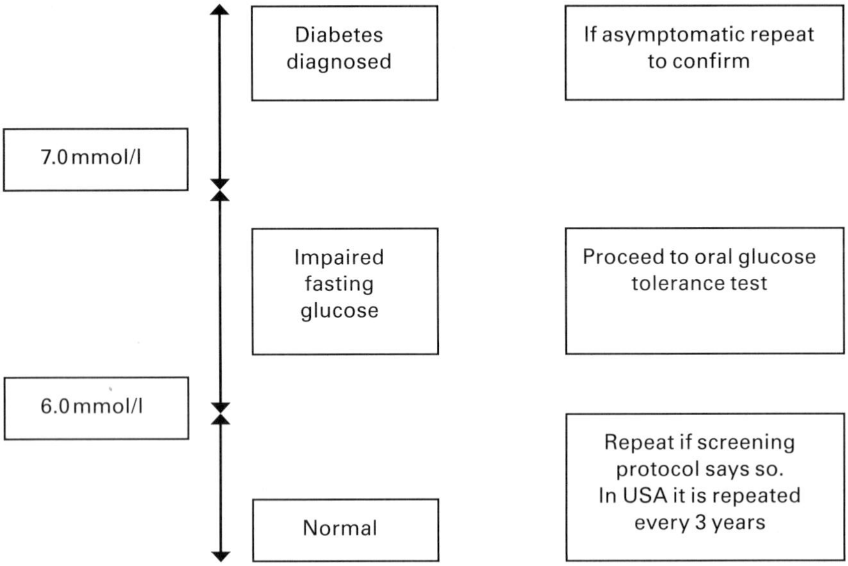

Source: Gadsby R. *Delivering Quality Diabetes Care in General Practice.*[3]

On random or post-glucose challenge results

The blood glucose level for diagnosing diabetes on a random plasma glucose or a 2-hour post-75 g glucose challenge is 11.1 mmol and above (see Figure 2.2).

Figure 2.2 ○ *Oral glucose tolerance test*

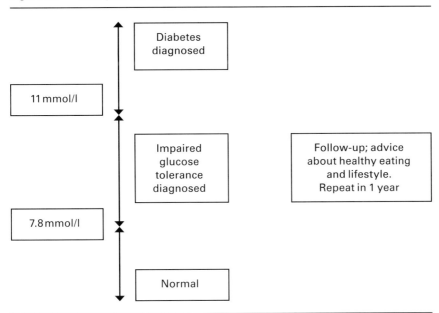

Source: Gadsby R. *Delivering Quality Diabetes Care in General Practice.*[3]

In asymptomatic people

Two abnormal blood glucose measurements diagnostic of diabetes must be obtained.

Impaired fasting glucose

Under these new criteria those with fasting glucose levels below 6 mmol are classified as normal and those with levels between 6 and 7 are classified as having impaired fasting glucose (IFG).

If IFG is diagnosed, Diabetes UK recommends that an oral glucose tolerance test (OGTT) is performed[2] to indicate if blood glucose levels are diagnostic of diabetes. To perform an OGTT a patient has a fasting blood specimen taken and is then given 75 g of glucose orally. A further blood glucose estimation is taken 2 hours later.

If the 2-hour glucose level is 11.1 or above diabetes is diagnosed. If the 2-hour level is below 7.8 it is classified as normal, and if it is between 7.8 and 11.1 a diagnosis of impaired glucose tolerance (IGT) is made.

These points are illustrated in Figure 2.2.

The diagnosis of diabetes has important medico-legal implications, e.g. for driving and insurance, so diagnostic blood glucose estimations must be from a laboratory with appropriate quality control mechanisms, rather than measurements of glucose obtained from a home blood glucose monitor.

Treating people with IGT and IFG

Those newly diagnosed with abnormal glycaemia involving IFG and/or IGT need a full CHD risk assessment and management of risk factors. They are at an increased risk of CHD as compared with people with normoglycaemia, but not such a great risk as those diagnosed with frank diabetes. Advice about weight loss and increased exercise should be given as these interventions have been shown to reduce the risk of developing diabetes.

Summary point

▶ Patients should have an annual measure of glycaemia to ensure that they have not developed frank diabetes. An annual fasting glucose estimation is the easiest to obtain.

Scenario 1 revisited

In discussion with Margaret you decide to request an OGTT. The results show a fasting level of 6.3 mmol/l and a 2-hour post-glucose load level of 10.6 mmol/l.

The diagnosis therefore is IGT and IFG.

Her CHD risks have been evaluated and she is on an ACE inhibitor and a statin.

You discuss weight loss, healthy eating and increasing her physical activity levels with her, and plan to repeat a fasting glucose level in a year. You put her on the practice register of people with IFG/IGT to ensure follow-up occurs.

Scenario 2

George is a 9-year-old boy who is brought to see you by his mother. She is worried that he has been getting very thirsty for the past 2 weeks and thinks that he has lost about 5 lbs in weight over the last month. He has had some abdominal pain and has vomited once or twice a day for the past 3 days. On direct questioning

George says he has been waking up at night for the past week to have a drink of water. George looks reasonably well on examination and does not look dehydrated.

His urine shows +++ of glucose, and ++ of ketones. A finger prick blood glucose reading done in the surgery is 18.9 mmol/l.

▶ *How would you manage George?*

Type 1 diabetes – definition

In Type 1 diabetes there is an absolute lack of insulin, which is caused by autoimmune destruction of beta cells in the pancreas. The exact aetiology of this autoimmune destruction is complex and not well understood. Some unknown environmental factor triggers this autoimmune process in individuals with an inherited predisposition.

Epidemiology

Information from studies in the UK suggests that there has been an increase in the incidence of diabetes in the under-16 age group from 16.5 to 19 per 100,000 children per year from 1991 to 1998. This is predicted to rise to 27 per 100,000 in 2005 and to 30 in 2010. Incidence is higher in boys than girls, and is highest in the more northerly parts of the UK. This increase in childhood diabetes is a consistent finding in most paediatric diabetes registers in the UK and other countries.[4]

There is a wide variation in the prevalence of Type 1 diabetes in different countries across the world. There is a 40-fold difference in reported prevalence of Type 1 diabetes in Finland (the country with the highest prevalence) and Japan (a country with one of the lowest reported prevalence rates).[5]

Costs to the NHS

The NICE guideline for adults[6] with Type 1 diabetes estimates NHS expenditure to be £212 million at 2001 prices, and includes costs of:

▷ £38 million for renal replacement therapy
▷ £50 million for out-patient support costs
▷ £65 million for hospitalisation.

Presentation

Type 1 diabetes typically presents after a short history (typically a few days or weeks) of thirst, polyuria and weight loss. This is often accompanied by nausea, vomiting, abdominal pain and dehydration.

Diagnosis

Type 1 diabetes is confirmed by a single diagnostic (i.e. above 11.1 mmol/l in a random sample) laboratory blood glucose measurement in the presence of classical symptoms, or by a further diagnostic blood glucose measurement. The diagnosis may be supported by a raised Hb_{A1c} level.

Where diabetes is diagnosed, but Type 2 diabetes suspected, the diagnosis of Type 1 diabetes should be considered if ketonuria is detected, or weight loss is marked, or the patient does not have features of the metabolic syndrome or other contributing illness.

Where diabetes is diagnosed in a child or teenager, the presence of obesity or a family history of Type 2 diabetes, especially in someone of non-white ethnicity, should suggest the possibility that the diabetes is not Type 1.

It is not usually necessary to detect specific auto-antibodies or measure c-peptide deficiency to diagnose Type 1 diabetes, although in certain circumstances they may be useful in distinguishing Type 1 from Type 2 diabetes.

Initial management and referral

If a patient presents in primary care with symptoms suggestive of Type 1 diabetes, a urine check for glycosuria and ketonuria and a finger prick blood glucose test should be carried out immediately. The presence of glycosuria, ketonuria and a raised blood glucose are very suggestive. A definitive diagnosis can be made if a laboratory blood glucose level is above 11.1 mmol/l.

Some people newly presenting with Type 1 diabetes have signs and symptoms suggestive of ketoacidosis, and if they are dehydrated and unwell immediate admission to a medical ward may be needed.

Others may have only mild symptoms, but a laboratory blood glucose measurement needs to be performed straight away. If this is diagnostic of Type 1 diabetes, referral to the local diabetes team for assessment and initiation of insulin treatment as an out-patient needs to be made immediately.

If the person newly presenting with Type 1 diabetes is a child or a young person, referral will need to be made to the paediatric diabetes service.

The NICE guideline for children and young people states that at the time of diagnosis they should be offered home-based or in-patient management according to clinical need, family circumstances and wishes. It states that home-based care with support from the local paediatric diabetes care team (including 24-hour telephone access to advice) is as safe and effective as in-patient initial management.[7]

Education

Both the adult and the younger person's NICE guideline on Type 1 diabetes[7] stress the need for initial and ongoing education. The adult guideline states that culturally appropriate education should be offered after diagnosis to all adults with Type 1 diabetes (and to those with significant input into the diabetes care of others). It should be repeated as requested and according to annual review of need. This should encompass the necessary understanding, motivation and skills to manage appropriately:[6]

▷ blood glucose control (insulin, self-monitoring, nutrition)
▷ arterial risk factors (blood lipids, blood pressure, smoking)
▷ late complications (feet, kidneys, eyes, heart).

Initial education will be given by the secondary care-based diabetes team. Some people with well-controlled Type 1 diabetes may choose to have their routine care in general practice, and education can then be reinforced at the annual review visit.

The **d**ose **a**djustment **f**or **n**ormal **e**ating (DAFNE) training and education programme is initially for adults with Type 1 diabetes in the UK. It enables participants to adjust their dose of insulin depending on their self-monitoring of blood glucose results, the type and size of meal they are going to eat, and the amount of exercise they are going to do. It enables patients with Type 1 diabetes to have a more flexible lifestyle, and has been shown to improve glycaemic control.[8] The programme is now being rolled out across the UK and should be available in local diabetes centres.

As children with Type 1 diabetes become adolescents they need to move from diabetes care provided by paediatricians to care from adult diabetologists. Adolescence is sometimes a time of rebellion and diabetes control may deteriorate. The diabetes National Service Framework recommends in standard 6 that:[9, 10]

All young people with diabetes will experience a smooth transition of care from paediatric diabetes services to adult diabetes services, whether hospital or community-based,

*either directly or via a young people's clinic. The transition will be organised in part-
nership with each individual and at an age appropriate to and agreed with them.*

One model of a young persons' clinic (sometimes called a transitional care
clinic) is that of an informal clinic, usually run as a group in the evenings.
Here paediatric staff and adult diabetes staff can together interact and support teenagers with Type 1 diabetes.

Some teenagers disengage with specialist services during adolescence and
become lost to follow-up. They do however still need to acquire their repeat
prescriptions for insulin. They may well also attend the practice for intercur-
rent illnesses and medication review appointments. They may also attend
the practice nurse for immunisations and contraception advice. All of these
contacts are opportunities to try and re-engage with them. Some practice
computer systems allow messages to be placed on the notes so that when
the person attends, say for an immunisation, the fact that he or she has not
attended out-patient follow-up can be highlighted. Practice staff can then
gently explore the reasons for disengagement and encourage attendance. If
adolescents do not want to attend the hospital clinic they may be persuaded
to attend the practice diabetes clinic.

Blood glucose control

Blood glucose control in adults with Type 1 diabetes should be optimised
towards attaining Diabetes Control and Complications Trial-harmonised
glycosalated haemoglobin HbA_{1c} targets. For prevention of microvascular
disease this is less than 7.5 per cent, and for macrovascular disease less than
or equal to 6.5 per cent. The following should also be taken into account:

1 ▷ the experiences and preferences of the insulin user, in order to
avoid hypoglycaemia
2 ▷ the necessity to seek advice from professionals knowledgeable
about the range of available mealtime and basal insulins, and
about good combinations thereof and their optimal use.[11]

Children and young people with Type 1 diabetes and their families should
be informed that the target for long-term glycaemic control is an HbA_{1c} level
of less than 7.5 per cent without frequent disabling hypoglycaemia. Their
care package should be designed to attempt to achieve this.[7]

Insulin doses will need to be adjusted to achieve these levels of blood glucose control. Multiple insulin injection regimens (short-acting insulin three
times a day with meals and long-acting insulin at night), in people who prefer

them, should be used as part of an integrated package of which education, food and skills training should be integral parts. This can allow alterations of insulin dose depending on size and timing of meals, and can give much more freedom to eat more normally.

Insulin treatment

Unless insulin replacement is given, the severe insulin deficiency of Type 1 diabetes will result in hyperglycaemia, ketoacidosis and death. Insulin treatment is therefore given immediately in the newly diagnosed.

Types of insulin

The majority of people today use human-sequence insulin. It is manufactured using recombinant DNA technology in which the human insulin genes are inserted into yeast or bacteria cells, which can be grown in bulk and the 'human' insulin harvested from the cells. Porcine and bovine insulin, extracted and purified from animal pancreas, is still available for those who need it.

Insulin analogues are modified forms of human-sequence insulin produced by alterations or substitutions of specific amino acids. The analogue insulins produced may be 'long acting' or 'rapid acting'. See the specific sections later.

There are several types of insulin.

1 ▷ short- and longer-acting traditional insulins, and mixtures of these
2 ▷ rapid- and long-acting analogue insulins, and mixtures of rapid-acting analogues and traditional long-acting insulins.

Short-acting insulin

These are known as clear or soluble insulins. They have a peak action 2 to 6 hours after injection. They should be given 20 to 30 minutes before meals. One of the best known examples is Human Actrapid.

Longer-acting insulins

These are cloudy insulins. They are made by precipitating insulin or protamine-insulin (neutral protamine Hagedorn (NPH) insulins, named after the person who invented them) in the presence of zinc. This forms insoluble crystals that are injected as a suspension and absorbed slowly. These insulins have a peak action at around 8 hours after injection, but in some people their effect can last for up to 18 hours.

Pre-mixed insulins

These contain combinations of soluble, short-acting and crystalline long-acting insulin. A combination of 30 per cent short acting and 70 per cent long acting is one that is often used, but 10:90, 15:85, 20:80, 25:75, 40:60 and 50:50 combinations are produced by different companies.

Rapid-acting insulin analogues

These have been developed by minor alterations to the amino acid sequence of human insulin to produce insulins that have a quicker onset of action and shorter duration of action than normal soluble insulin. Three are available:

▷ insulin lispro, which is identical to human insulin apart from inversion of lysine and proline residues at positions B28 and B29 on the B chain of the insulin molecule
▷ insulin aspart, which is identical to human insulin apart from the substitution of proline at position B28 with aspartic acid
▷ insulin glulisine.

These three short-acting analogues have similar pharmacokinetic profiles, with quicker onset and shorter duration of action than traditional soluble insulin. Their peak action is around 1 hour after injection and their effect wanes after 4 hours. This means that they can be injected just before a meal, and they reduce the risk of postprandial hypoglycaemia.[11]

They are now available pre-mixed with longer-acting cloudy insulins, in varying combinations for those using a twice-daily pre-mixed regime.

Long-acting insulin analogues

Two long-acting insulin analogues have been developed and marketed. One, insulin glargine, is the same as human insulin apart from a substitution of glycine for asparagine at the A chain of the insulin molecule at position A21 and the addition of two arginine molecules at the C terminal end of the B chain. This results in a change in properties of insulin glargine. It is soluble at acidic pH and so is the first clear long-acting insulin. When it is injected it forms a micro-precipitate within the more neutral pH of the subcutaneous tissues. This results in slow absorption from the injection site. It has a flat profile of action with no pronounced peaks, has a duration of action of around 24 hours and is subject to less inter- and intra-person variability than previous cloudy long-acting insulins. As a result there is often a reduction in hypoglycaemic episodes in people using insulin glargine as compared with NPH insulin.[12]

The other, insulin detemir, is acylated with a fatty acid at the C terminus of the insulin B chain. The fatty acid binds to albumin, which slows insulin absorption and prolongs the circulation time. Insulin detemir has a flat profile of action, and reduces the number of hypoglycaemic episodes as compared with long-acting cloudy NPH insulins.[13]

Insulin delivery systems

Most insulins are available in 10 ml vials, pen cartridges and disposable pens. A good analogy is that of pen and writing. Vials are like dipping a quill into ink, insulin cartridges are like cartridge pens, and disposable pens are biros! Pen technology enables insulin to be carried about easily and enables injections to be given where and when required. Insulin doses can be dialled up more accurately using the pen devices, and it is easier to teach people to use pen devices than it is to draw up insulin into a syringe from a vial. Most people moving on to insulin when offered a choice prefer pen devices and they are now commonly being prescribed for initiation of insulin in both Type 1 and Type 2 diabetes. Some healthcare professionals prefer cartridges and others the disposable pens. Patient choice should inform the decision as to which to use.

A few people with Type 1 diabetes use continuous infusion pumps, which give a slow, steady infusion of short-acting insulin. Pump technology has developed significantly in the past few years. However, it is expensive and there are limited NHS funds for it. Such people will be under the care of a secondary or tertiary diabetes care centre.

Advice about insulin injections

Insulin needles are nowadays very thin and short, enabling the injection to be almost 'pain free'. Insulin is usually injected at right angles into the subcutaneous tissue of the lower abdomen or the upper outer thighs. The upper outer arms or buttocks can also be used if necessary. Repeated injection into the same site can cause accumulation of fat (called lipohypertrophy). This can be a cosmetic embarrassment and can cause variability in the absorption of insulin. Injection sites should therefore be rotated to avoid this possible complication.

Insulin regimes

Basal bolus therapy is the insulin regime in which an injection of short-acting insulin is given just before each meal, with one injection of long-acting insulin at night. People using this regime usually have four injections a day. It gives flexibility to cope with different meal times, size of meals and exercise.

Another regime is to have two daily injections of pre-mixed insulin, one before breakfast and the other before the evening meal. Some children may initially manage on one injection of long-acting insulin each day.

The variety of different insulins available is considerable and can make prescribing complex. This is one reason why insulin treatment has been the territory of the specialist rather than the GP. It is important to understand these paragraphs as you may be required to adjust insulin dosages and issue repeat prescriptions.

Type 1 diabetes and the Quality and Outcomes Framework

People with Type 1 diabetes have traditionally received most of their routine follow-up in secondary care. Results from their secondary care clinic attendance will therefore arrive in letters to the practice. These results will need to be put on the practice's clinical computer system, as these patients are included in all the Quality and Outcomes Framework (QoF) clinical indicators for diabetes.

A number of people with Type 1 diabetes disengage from follow-up during the teenage years. They may occasionally attend primary care, but often this is only for acute illness unrelated to diabetes. It is vital to try to re-engage with them and every opportunity needs to be taken to discuss their diabetes and its control. As the responsibility for issuing prescriptions for insulin falls to primary care, repeat prescription monitoring may offer an opportunity to renew contact with these patients and the chance to discuss their care.

Scenario 2 revisited

George presents with most of the features of Type 1 diabetes.

You phone the local paediatric diabetes team, who arranges to see George that afternoon.

Laboratory blood tests confirm an elevated blood glucose; Type 1 diabetes is confirmed. He and his parents are taught self-monitoring of blood glucose and how to give insulin injections. He is started on an analogue mixed insulin b.d., and the diabetes team see him every few days to adjust his insulin dose.

George quickly feels much better on insulin. His parents learn to give him the insulin injections and to carry out self-monitoring of blood glucose (SMBG).

Summary

In relation to the six domains of core or essential competences of being a GP:

1 Primary care management

▷ Recognising the signs and symptoms in newly presenting Type 1 diabetes.
▷ Understanding the diagnosis of diabetes and the categories of IGT and IFG, and how to manage these.
▷ Arranging appropriate annual testing of people with IFG or IGT to detect developing diabetes.
▷ Educating people with IGT or IFG about the steps they can take to reduce their risk of developing diabetes.

2 Person-centred care

▷ Understanding the impact of a new diagnosis of Type 1 diabetes on the individual and how the responsibility for the management will need to transfer from the parents to the individual as the child grows.
▷ Being aware of the difficulties a number of children with Type 1 diabetes can have during teenage years and how they can be supported.
▷ Similarly, for Type 2 diabetes, being aware of the need for changes in lifestyle including diet and treatment of other risk factors such as lipids.

3 Specific problem-solving skills

▷ Being able to support and help someone with Type 1 diabetes to navigate from paediatric care to adult diabetes care, hopefully through a period in an adolescent/transitional clinic.
▷ Remembering the possibility of the diagnosis of an older person who is tired and unwell.

4 A comprehensive approach

▷ Understanding the effect that Type 1 diabetes will have on teenagers in respect of issues of sex, drinking alcohol, going out for meals, and giving themselves injections.

5 Community orientation

▷ Encouraging the individual to get support and help from others with diabetes by attending the local Diabetes UK support group.
▷ Understanding the epidemiology and costs to the NHS of Type 1 diabetes and its treatment.
▷ For patients on insulin, understanding the importance of advising about the rules and regulations concerning driving and the DVLA.

6 A holistic approach

▷ Understanding the impact that Type 1 diabetes has on the individual and his or her life, and similarly for the patient with Type 2 diabetes on, for example, his or her work and driving.

References

1 • World Health Organization. *Definition, Diagnosis and Classification of Diabetes Mellitus and its Complications: report of a WHO consultation. Part 1: diagnosis and classification of diabetes mellitus* Geneva: WHO, 1999.

2 • Diabetes UK. *Recommendations for the Management of Diabetes in Primary Care* (second edn) London: Diabetes UK, 2006.

3 • Gadsby R. *Delivering Quality Diabetes Care in General Practice* London: RCGP, 2005.

4 • Gadsby R. Epidemiology of diabetes *Advanced Drug Delivery Reviews* 2002; **54**: 1165–72.

5 • Karvonen M, Tuomilehto J, Libman I, *et al*. A review of the recent epidemiological data on the worldwide incidence of type 1 diabetes mellitus *Diabetologia* 1993; **36(10)**: 883–92.

6 • National Institute for Health and Clinical Excellence. *Type 1 Diabetes: management of type 1 diabetes in adults* London: NICE, 2004, www.nice.org.uk.

7 • National Institute for Health and Clinical Excellence. *Type 1 Diabetes: diagnosis and management of type 1 diabetes in children and young people* London: NICE, 2004, www.nice.org.uk.

8 • Amiel S, Beveridge S, Bradley C, *et al*. Training in flexible, intensive insulin management to enable dietary freedom in people with type 1 diabetes: dose adjustment for normal eating (DAFNE) randomised controlled trial *British Medical Journal* 2002; **325**: 746–9.

9 • Department of Health. *National Service Framework for Diabetes: standards* London: DoH, 2001, www.dh.gov.uk/en/Publicationsandstatistics/Publications/ PublicationsPolicyAndGuidance/DH_4003246 [accessed July 2009].

10 • Department of Health. *National Service Framework for Diabetes: delivery strategy* London: DoH, 2002, www.dh.gov.uk/en/Publicationsandstatistics/Publications/ PublicationsPolicyAndGuidance/DH_4003246 [accessed July 2009].

11 • Oiknine R, Bernbaum M, Mooradian A D. A critical appraisal of the role of insulin analogues in the management of diabetes mellitus *Drugs* 2005; **65(3)**: 325–40.

12 • Hamann A, Matthaei S, Rosak C, *et al.* A randomized clinical trial comparing breakfast, dinner or bedtime administration of insulin glargine in patients with type 1 diabetes *Diabetes Care* 2003; **26**: 1738–44.

13 • Vague P, Selam J L, Skeie S, *et al.* Insulin detemir is associated with more predictable glycaemic control and reduced risk of hypoglycaemia than NPH insulin in patients with type 1 diabetes on a basal-bolus regime with premeal insulin aspart *Diabetes Care* 2003; **26**: 590–6.

Managing acute diabetes problems

3

Scenario 1

You are in the middle of a normal morning surgery when you get a call from reception asking if you would go straight away to the practice nurses' room to see a patient, Peter, who has collapsed. Peter arrived a few minutes before his diabetes clinic appointment, had felt unwell in the waiting room and collapsed. You learn from his notes that he is a 63-year-old man who has had Type 2 diabetes for 13 years and is currently being treated with metformin and twice-daily mixed insulin.

▶ *You find Peter lying on a couch in the nurses' room. He is sweaty and unconscious, and has a pounding pulse.*

What is the likely diagnosis and how would you confirm this?

The examination findings suggest that hypoglycaemia is likely to be the cause of the 'collapse'. This can be confirmed by getting a finger-prick glucose estimation done immediately. It is 1.5 mmol/l.

What is the immediate treatment for this patient?

IV glucose is the treatment of choice in this situation. Twenty millilitres of 25 per cent glucose is given through a wide-bore needle into a large vein. The best site for the injection is usually the ante-cubital fossa and help will be needed to keep the patient's arm straight to ensure that no glucose leaks into the tissues.

Hypoglycaemia – how common is it?

Incidence rates for severe hypoglycaemia (defined as hypoglycaemia of such severity as to require help from healthcare personnel) in a Scottish community survey were 11.5 and 11.8 events per 100 patient years in Type 1 and Type 2 diabetes treated with insulin. In the study period 7.1 per cent of people with Type 1 diabetes, 7.3 per cent with Type 2 treated with insulin, and 0.8 per cent with Type 2 treated with a sulphonylurea had a severe hypoglycaemic episode. Age, duration of diabetes and socioeconomic status were identified as risk factors for severe hypoglycaemia.[1]

It is important to note that rates of hypoglycaemia are not normally distributed. In surveys of individuals with either Type 1 or Type 2 diabetes a small proportion experience a large number of episodes whilst many experience no episodes at all.[2]

What symptoms can occur?

Symptoms are classified into two groups, autonomic and neuroglycopenic.

Autonomic ones are those due to activation of the sympathetic or parasympathetic nervous system, and consist of:

▷ sweating
▷ a pounding heart
▷ shakiness or tremor
▷ hunger.

Neuroglycopenic ones are those due to the effects of glucose deprivation on the brain. They consist of:

▷ confusion
▷ drowsiness
▷ difficulty with speech
▷ incoordination.

A mixture of autonomic and neuroglycopenic symptoms usually occur together. The partners and carers of people with diabetes who experience frequent hypoglycaemia events often become aware of impending hypoglycaemia as the patient develops subtle cognitive changes (e.g. hesitation in speech). Once recognised the patient can be encouraged to take oral glucose before more severe symptoms develop.

At what level of blood glucose does hypoglycaemia occur?

In non-diabetic subjects release of glucagon and catecholamines, hormones that raise blood glucose, occurs at arterial plasma glucose levels of around 3.8 mmol/l. Autonomic symptoms develop at about 3.2 mmol/l and cognitive function starts to deteriorate at around 3.0 mmol/l. People who have normal

awareness of hypoglycaemia therefore get symptoms and can take correc-
tive action before significant cerebral dysfunction occurs.

Treating hypoglycaemia

The management of hypoglycaemia depends on the level of consciousness
and co-operation.

If the person is conscious and co-operative

1 ▷ Give a sugary drink, e.g. glass of milk with four spoons of sugar
in it, or three or four glucose sweets.
2 ▷ Follow this with a substantial snack or meal high in carbohydrate.
3 ▷ Check blood glucose levels to ensure that they have returned to
normal.

If the person is conscious but uncooperative

Use dextrose gel (GlucoGel). Insert the gel into the mouth, using around a
third of the bottle, and massage gently around the cheeks to aid absorption
of the gel through the buccal mucosa. Then repeat steps 1 to 3 above.

If the person is unconscious

Give a subcutaneous (SC) or intramuscular (IM) glucagon injection. Place
the person in the recovery position and await the return of consciousness,
which usually occurs in 15 to 20 minutes.

If glucagon doesn't render the person conscious

Contact an ambulance. Paramedics or medical personnel can then give an
IV injection of glucose, usually in the form of 20 ml of 25 per cent or 50 per
cent glucose solution given into a large vein through a wide-bore needle.

Great caution is needed with venous access as concentrated glucose solu-
tions can damage tissue if they leak out of a vein, so care must be taken to
ensure that this does not occur.

What is hypoglycaemic unawareness?

Hypoglycaemic unawareness is when an individual who has diabetes loses the early warning signs of impending hypoglycaemia. Individuals with hypoglycaemic unawareness can go from feeling normal to profound hypoglycaemia without symptomatic warning, and therefore are unable to take any action to alleviate the problem.

People who have hypoglycaemic unawareness may have significant problems with driving, and should be told not to drive until the condition is reversed.

Unawareness increases with duration of diabetes, in situations of repeated hypoglycaemia, where there is autonomic neuropathy and in situations of intensive glycaemic control. It can often be reversed, at least in part, by strict avoidance of hypoglycaemia.

What causes hypoglycaemia?

Hypoglycaemia can only occur in people with diabetes being treated with agents that can lower blood glucose. These are insulin and oral agents that cause insulin secretion such as sulphonylureas. Hypoglycaemia does not occur in people with diabetes treated with diet and/or metformin and glitazones. Hypoglycaemia occurs in people with diabetes who are on insulin or sulphonylureas when there is a raised insulin concentration or enhanced insulin effect.

Raised insulin concentrations can occur when a diabetic patient or healthcare professional gives too much insulin in error. Here there is a mismatch between the insulin dose and a patient's needs or lifestyle, through a deliberate overdose, or through accelerated absorption of insulin (e.g. in hot weather).

The usual reasons for an enhanced insulin effect are increased physical activity and delayed or missed meals.

It is important to find out the cause of any episode of hypoglycaemia to try to avoid a repeat in the future.

Scenario 1 revisited

Peter regains consciousness within 30 seconds of the IV glucose injection. He is then given four biscuits to eat. Peter is asked about the events before he got to the surgery this morning. He says that he had his normal insulin injection at breakfast but discovered he was running late for his diabetes clinic appointment. He only half-finished his breakfast and had to run to catch the bus. He then had a very brisk 10 minute walk to the surgery from the bus stop. He felt rather sweaty in the waiting room and then felt faint and drowsy. He tried to get a glucose sweet out of his pocket but felt himself collapsing. The next thing he remembers is waking up in the nurses' room.

It seems clear that the cause of Peter's hypoglycaemic episode was not taking enough breakfast combined with the extra physical activity of running for the bus and walking briskly to the surgery. The lessons about eating enough food and taking extra glucose if extra physical activity is to be undertaken need to be reinforced to try to ensure that Peter avoids getting a similar episode in the future.

Diabetic ketoacidosis

Scenario 2

Susan is a 19-year-old woman who has had Type 1 diabetes for 10 years. She takes a short-acting insulin injection before each of her three meals and an injection of long-acting insulin at night. She comes to your afternoon surgery complaining of dysuria and frequency for 2 days and a 1-day history of vomiting and abdominal pain. She looks unwell and is slightly dehydrated.

What are the likely diagnoses and how would you confirm these?

It is likely that Susan has a urinary tract infection (UTI). This can be confirmed by dip testing a urine sample. It is possible that this infection is causing her to become ketoacidotic. It is important therefore to check the urine sample for ketones and to check her blood glucose level. She looks clinically dehydrated.

Dip stick testing of the urine shows 2+ of leucocytes and protein. There are also 3+ of ketones. Her finger-prick test blood glucose is 25.3 mmol/l.

What action needs to be taken?

Susan has diabetic ketoacidosis (DKA) and needs immediate admission to hospital for treatment to correct her dehydration and ketoacidosis. On admission she is assessed and treated according to the hospital DKA protocol.

Definition and epidemiology

DKA is defined as a combination of hyperglycaemia, ketonuria and a serum bicarbonate of below 15 mmol/l. The risk of DKA in established Type 1 diabetes is 1–10 per cent per patient per year.[3] Risk is increased in peripubertal and adolescent girls, people with psychiatric disorders (including eating disorders), people with poor metabolic control and a history of previous episodes of DKA, and people on insulin pump therapy (as only rapid-acting or short-acting insulin is used in pumps, interruption of insulin delivery for whatever reason rapidly leads to insulin deficiency and DKA).

Causes of diabetic ketoacidosis

The causes of DKA are:

▷ omitting insulin injections
▷ previously undiagnosed Type 1 diabetes (around 25 per cent of people with newly diagnosed diabetes present with DKA)
▷ infection, e.g. UTI, chest infection, etc.

Signs and symptoms of diabetic ketoacidosis

In DKA the symptoms are thirst, polyuria, weight loss, weakness, nausea, leg cramps, drowsiness and eventually coma. Abdominal pain may occur.

Signs include dehydration, hypotension, tachycardia, hyperventilation and a sweet smell on the breath.

Treatment of diabetic ketoacidosis

Urgent admission is necessary for assessment and management. The principles of management include:

1 ▷ restoration of blood volume with intravenous fluids, usually normal saline
2 ▷ restoration of insulin, usually by low-dose continuous insulin infusion
3 ▷ controlling potassium concentrations by regular monitoring and IV potassium infusion as needed.

Hospitals will have a DKA protocol giving detailed instructions as to how to implement the above principles. An excellent summary of the principles of DKA management is contained in the Consensus Guidelines of the International Society for Paediatric and Adolescent Diabetes.[4]

Scenario 2 revisited

Susan made a good recovery from her episode of DKA. She spent 1 day in Intensive Treatment Unit (ITU) and 4 days on a normal ward before discharge. Her UTI was successfully treated with antibiotics. Before admission her diabetes control had been suboptimal so before discharge she had a one-to-one diabetes education session with the diabetes specialist nurse (DSN), which helped her to think about ways to improve her glycaemic control. The importance of early treatment of UTIs was stressed as well as the need to try to maintain fluid intake during infections.

Hyperosmolar non-ketotic state

Scenario 3

Bill is a 69-year-old man who has had Type 2 diabetes for 16 years. He is treated with metformin 500 mg 2 tablets b.d. and gliclazide 80 mg b.d. He came to see you in the surgery 10 days ago with a chest infection for which you prescribed amoxicillin 500 mg t.d.s. for 7 days. He attends today feeling tired and thirsty, with a productive cough. On examination he looks very ill and dehydrated, with a tachycardia of 110 and right basal chest signs.

What is the likely diagnosis and how would you confirm this?

The chest signs indicate a right-sided basal bronchopneumonia. The fact that he looks so ill and dehydrated suggests that he may be significantly hyperglycaemic. A finger-prick blood glucose registers high. A urine sample contains no ketones.

What is the immediate treatment for this patient?

Bill needs to be admitted to hospital as an emergency. He has signs of a bronchopneumonia and is very hyperglycaemic (high on a finger-prick meter usually means blood glucose levels of above 33 mmol/l). He does not have ketonuria and so the probable diagnosis is hyperosmolar non-ketotic state (HONK), which is called hyperosmolar hyperglycaemic state (HHS) in the USA.

Definition and epidemiology

HONK is defined as the combination of hyperglycaemia (the blood glucose level is often above 50 mmol/l) and hyperosmolality (usually above 330 mosmol/kg) without ketonuria. The absence of ketones is incompletely explained, but may involve the preservation of endogenous insulin production that occurs in Type 2 diabetes, and the suppression of lipolysis by hyperosmolality. Certain ethnic groups, particularly Afro-Caribbean patients, are thought to have a higher risk. Although it is a relatively uncommon cause of hospital admissions (around 1 per cent) it has a fairly high mortality rate of around 15 per cent in a recent series.[5] Death is most commonly due to sepsis, although thrombo-embolic complications are also common.

Causes

Precipitating causes of HONK include infection and other causes of metabolic derangement including myocardial infarction.

Signs and symptoms

Signs and symptoms are increasing tiredness, lethargy and eventually coma, thirst and signs of dehydration. Patients may have raised creatinine concentrations reflecting prerenal uraemia, but acute renal failure may sometimes accompany HONK, especially after prolonged dehydration and hypotension.

Treatment

Immediate admission to hospital is needed for assessment and management. Treatment is similar to that of DKA. However, fluid deficit is often greater than in DKA, but patients with HONK are often elderly and have significant co-morbidities, so infusion rates need to be carefully monitored. The fluid of choice is 0.9 per cent saline, although if serum sodium concentrations rise some authorities recommend 0.45 per cent saline. Insulin should be given by low-dose continuous infusion at similar rates as in DKA. Some also recommend giving low molecular weight heparin to prevent venous thrombosis.[6]

Scenario 3 revisited

Bill recovered from his admission for HONK precipitated by bronchopneumonia, but he had to stay in hospital for 3 weeks. He was in ITU for 5 days. He was discharged on a basal bolus insulin regime, but after 3 months he was able to be transferred back onto the oral agent regime he was on before admission.

Summary

In relation to the six domains of core or essential competences of being a GP:

1 Primary care management

▷ Recognition and management of hypoglycaemia, diabetic ketoacidosis and hyperosmolar non-ketotic state.

2 Person-centred care

▷ Understanding the precipitating factors in an individual that could have led to an acute diabetes complication, and how those factors may be modified to prevent the acute complications happening again.

3 Specific problem-solving skills

▷ Managing the co-morbidities in older people with diabetes to prevent hyperglycaemic complications.

4 A comprehensive approach

▷ Appropriate recognition and emergency referral of people with acute diabetes complications that need hospital treatment.
▷ Liaison with ambulance staff and secondary care to ensure appropriate pre-hospital management and safe transfer.

5 Community orientation

▷ Educating patients with diabetes at risk of developing acute complications that it is important to carry identification and information about their diabetes at all times. Thus, if hypoglycaemia symptoms develop, those around them can identify the symptoms and offer help.

6 A holistic approach

▷ Understanding the psychological impact of acute complications.
▷ Giving appropriate support and encouragement to those who have experienced acute complications.

References

1 • Leese G, Wang J, Broomhall J, *et al.* Frequency of severe hypoglycaemia requiring emergency treatment in type 1 and type 2 diabetes *Diabetes Care* 2003; **26**: 1176–80.

2 • Heller S. Acute complications: hypoglycaemia. In: AJ Barnett (ed.) *Diabetes Best Practice and Research Compendium* Philadelphia: Elsevier, 2006, p.64.

3 • Rewers A, Chase HP, Mackenzie T, *et al.* Predictors of acute complications in children with type 1 diabetes *Journal of the American Medical Association* 2002; **287**: 2511–18.

4 • Wolfsdorf J, Craig MA, Daneman D, *et al.* Diabetic ketoacidosis *Paediatric Diabetes* 2007; **8**: 28–42.

5 • Pinies JA, Cairo C, Gaztambide S, *et al.* Course and prognosis of 132 patients with diabetic non ketotic hyperosmolar state *Diabète & métabolisme* 1994; **20**: 43–8.

6 • Heller SR. Acute complications in diabetes. In: AJ Barnett (ed.) *Diabetes Best Practice and Research Compendium* Philadelphia: Elsevier, 2006, pp.71–2.

Treating glycaemia in Type 2 diabetes

4

Scenario

David is a 62-year-old patient who has had Type 2 diabetes for 9 years. He is taking the biguanide metformin 1 gm b.d. and the sulphonylurea gliclazide 160 mg b.d. He has no other co-morbidities. He is feeling a bit tired. His HbA1c, which was 7.1 per cent 6 months ago, has risen to 8.2 per cent. David has recently had lifestyle, diet and physical activity advice reinforced, and does not think he can do any more to improve this. His BMI is 26. He works as a bus driver and wants to continue till he is 65.

▶ *What treatment options are there to try to optimise his glycaemic control?*

Aims of treatment

There is high-quality evidence, in both Type 1 and Type 2 diabetes, that intensive control of blood glucose (giving Hb_{A1c} measurements of 7 per cent or less) reduces the risk of adverse outcomes.

Box 4.1 ○ **Evidence from trials that good glycaemic control reduces complications in Type 1 and Type 2 diabetes**

In Type 1 diabetes the evidence comes from the Diabetes Control and Complications Trial (DCCT), which randomised 1441 people with Type 1 diabetes aged between 16 and 39 years into two groups. One group was intensively controlled and had Hb_{A1c} measurements averaging 7 per cent, while the other group received standard care and had Hb_{A1c} levels averaging 9 per cent. They were followed up for an average of 6.5 years.

Intensive treatment reduced the risk of severe retinopathy by 47 per cent and the need for laser treatment by 56 per cent. It also reduced the risk of developing microalbuminuria by 54 per cent and the risk of neuropathy by 60 per cent.[1]

The groups were followed up after the trial finished. Once the intensive support in the trial ended, the glycaemic control in the intensive group deteriorated to an average Hb_{A1c} of 8 per cent. However, the glycaemic control in the standard treatment group improved to 8 per cent. The groups have been followed and a

---

Continued over

paper has been published with results of a further 6 years' follow-up, showing that the group who were intensively treated still had fewer complications and less carotid intima-media thickness, which is a marker for atherosclerosis.[2] The conclusion is that intensive control, even for a limited time, has long-term benefits in reducing microvascular complications and as a surrogate marker for macrovascular complications.

The evidence in Type 2 diabetes comes from the United Kingdom Prospective Diabetes Study (UKPDS), which took 5102 people with newly diagnosed Type 2 diabetes and treated them with diet and exercise for 3 months.

Then 4209 of these who were asymptomatic and had fasting plasma glucose levels between 6 and 15 mmol/l were randomised into an intensively treated group, who had an average Hb_{A1c} of 7.9 per cent, and a conventionally treated group, who had an average Hb_{A1c} of 7 per cent. Treatment was initially with sulphonylurea medications or insulin. Follow-up was on average for 12 years. The intensive group had a 12 per cent less risk of any diabetes-related adverse endpoint, 25 per cent fewer adverse microvascular endpoints and 16 per cent fewer myocardial infarctions (this figure for major macrovascular outcomes did not reach statistical significance).[3] Neither sulphonylurea nor insulin therapy showed any advantage over each other, but a group of obese patients randomised to metformin had substantially better macrovascular outcomes.[4]

This UKPDS glycaemic data have also been published in an epidemiological form in which it can be shown that adverse outcomes are reduced for any reduction in Hb_{A1c} level even if a target of 7 per cent is not reached, thus a reduction of Hb_{A1c} from 10 per cent to 9 per cent is of benefit.[5]

Measuring glycaemia

Hb_{A1c}

Hb_{A1c} levels reflect the glycaemia present over the preceding 6–10 weeks. Hb_{A1c} levels are used to monitor glycaemic control in people with diabetes every 6–12 months when they are stable and every 3 months when glucose-lowering medications have been changed.

Hb_{A1c} is formed by the non-enzymatic glycation of the beta chain of red-cell haemoglobin. The UKPDS used the same method of measuring Hb_{A1c} as did the DCCT study. Laboratory values of Hb_{A1c} reported in the UK are aligned to this DCCT assay. From 1 June 2009 the way in which Hb_{A1c} results are reported in the UK is changing, as a result of international agreement on the standardisation of Hb_{A1c} measurement. The new units for Hb_{A1c} will be expressed as mmol per mol of haemoglobin without glucose attached. A DCCT-aligned Hb_{A1c} level of 7 per cent will be 53 in the new units. Until 1 June 2011 both values for Hb_{A1c} will be reported. A guidance leaflet is available at www.diabetes.nhs.uk/reading-room/nhs-diabetes-publications/factsheets/downloads/hba1c_factsheets/hba1c_hcp_leaflet.pdf.

Self-monitoring of blood glucose

Patients with diabetes can self-monitor their blood glucose (SMBG) using one of the many monitors available in the UK. A very small amount of blood is obtained by a finger-prick, which is then drawn up into the monitor by capillary action. Glucose levels are then estimated by the monitor and given as a read-out, usually within a few seconds.

Patients using insulin, whether they have Type 1 or Type 2 diabetes, need to be able to monitor their blood glucose levels. Blood glucose monitoring enables them to vary doses of insulin according to the level of physical activity and eating pattern on a dose-by-dose basis. This gives much more flexibility in daily living and gives the opportunity for improved overall control.

In Type 2 diabetes treated with oral agents and/or diet alone, there is much less consensus about the benefits of blood glucose monitoring. A meta-analysis of studies on self-monitoring in Type 2 diabetes failed to demonstrate the effectiveness of blood glucose monitoring in improving glycaemic control, and failed to demonstrate a difference in diabetes control between blood and urine glucose monitoring.[6] A very recent randomised control trial in the UK has again failed to show that SMBG is of value in reducing Hb_{Alc} levels in people with Type 2 diabetes controlled by oral agents.[7]

In some areas of the UK spending on blood glucose monitoring now exceeds that of insulin itself, and attempts are being made to rationalise prescribing of blood glucose-testing sticks. However, it seems reasonable to support the argument that patients with diabetes who are using insulin should be prescribed enough sticks to test as often as they need to. A recent consensus report has suggested guidelines for the rational use of blood glucose monitoring in Type 1 and Type 2 diabetes.[8]

For patients with Type 2 diabetes treated with oral agents and/or diet there is an argument that if they regularly blood glucose monitor until their Hb_{Alc} stabilises they will more quickly learn the relationship between exercise, food intake and blood glucose levels than those people who choose not to monitor their blood glucose levels. SMBG is therefore an integral part of many education programmes for people newly diagnosed with Type 2 diabetes.

Table 4.1 ○ *Classes of glucose-lowering agents*

Class	Mechanism of action
Sulphonylureas and prandial glucose regulators	Stimulate pancreatic beta cells to release insulin
Biguanides	Decrease hepatic gluconeogenesis and increase peripheral glucose uptake
Thiazolidinediones (glitazones)	Interact with PPARγ to upregulate transcription of insulin-responsive genes
Alpha-glucosidase inhibitors	Delays absorption of glucose from gut
Incretins:	
GLP-1 mimetics	Increase GLP-1 levels
DPP-4 inhibitors	Reduce the breakdown of GLP-1

Insulin secretagogues (sulphonylureas and prandial glucose regulators)

There are six sulphonylureas available in the UK: glimepiride, glibenclamide, gliclazide, glipizide, gliquidone and tolbutamide. There are two short-acting insulin secretagogues, repaglinide and nateglinide.

They stimulate insulin release from the pancreatic beta cell, and are therefore dependent on the patient having adequate beta cell function. The main difference between members of the group is duration of action. Tolbutamide needs to be given three times a day, whilst the action of glibenclamide may last more than 24 hours. The prandial glucose regulators work within 10–30 minutes of ingestion and have a duration of action from 2 to 4 hours. They are given with each meal.

All insulin secretagogues effectively reduce glucose levels in monotherapy or in combination with metformin. It usually occurs within a few days, giving Hb$_{A1c}$ reductions of around 1 to 1.5 per cent.

They can be used as monotherapy if diet alone is insufficient, in thin people, and in those who have symptomatic hyperglycaemia when their rapid onset of action can be helpful in reducing symptoms quickly. They can be used with metformin in dual therapy. The short-acting agent repaglinide can be used in monotherapy or with metformin. Nateglinide can only be used with metformin. These short-acting agents are used with each meal, so they are useful if people have erratic eating patterns, e.g. shift workers.

The main side effects are hypoglycaemia and weight gain. Hypoglycaemia is more likely to occur with the longer-acting sulphonylureas, and gliben-

clamide should be avoided. Gliclazide has around 80 per cent of the sulphonylurea market in the UK.

Biguanides

Metformin is the only biguanide available in the UK. It inhibits hepatic
glucose production and enhances insulin-stimulated glucose uptake and
glycogenesis by skeletal muscle. Metformin improves some of the metabolic
actions of insulin and has additional beneficial effects independent of insulin. It does not stimulate insulin production.

Metformin lowers HbA_{1c} in line with all other oral agents, lowering HbA_{1c}
by 1–2 per cent. In the UKPDS study metformin had benefits over and above
its glycaemic-lowering effects to reduce adverse macrovascular outcomes.[4]
It is recommended as the initial monotherapy of choice in most people with
Type 2 diabetes, and is being given to some people with Type 1 diabetes for
its 'insulin-sparing' effect.

Metformin is excreted in the urine. The rare serious side effect associated
with metformin is lactic acidosis, and this can happen if metformin accu-
mulates in the body where there is renal impairment. Guidelines therefore
suggest not using metformin when the creatinine is above 130 mmol/l and
stopping metformin if the serum creatinine level rises above 150 mmol/l.

Metformin can give rise to gastrointestinal (GI) side effects of abdominal
pain, nausea, diarrhoea and a metallic taste in the mouth. Around 10–20
per cent do not continue on metformin because of these side effects. They
can be minimised by starting with a low dose, say 500 mg daily, and titrating up to 500 mg twice daily over 2 to 4 weeks. A once-daily formulation
of metformin has recently been released, and can be given as one to four
tablets once a day. It is said to cause fewer diarrhoea and GI side effects than
the generic preparation and should be considered where GI intolerability
prevents continuation of generic metformin therapy. Because of the risk of
lactic acidosis, metformin is contraindicated in people with uncontrolled
heart failure, renal failure and advanced liver disease.

Also, metformin is often given to overweight people with impaired glucose tolerance.

Thiazolidinediones

Two thiazolidinediones, or glitazones as they are more easily called, are
available in the UK. They are pioglitazone and rosiglitazone.

They work mainly by stimulating a nuclear receptor called peroxisome proliferator-activated receptor-gamma (PPARγ), which is most strongly expressed in adipose tissue. It acts to increase transcription of certain insulin-sensitive genes involved in the control of lipid and glucose metabolism. As a result they lower insulin resistance.

Glitazones produce a slowly generated blood glucose-lowering effect in Type 2 diabetes that may take 3 to 6 months to achieve maximal effect.

In combination treatment with metformin, glitazones lower HbA_{1c} in the range 0.6–1.2 per cent.

Glitazones are generally well tolerated. The main side effect is fluid retention with increased plasma volume, reduced haematocrit, and a decrease in haemoglobin. As a result, peripheral oedema, mainly at the ankles, may occur in some patients, and there is an increased association with congestive cardiac failure. There may be an associated weight gain of around 5 per cent. There is an increased risk of congestive cardiac failure but not of mortality from heart failure described in a recent systematic review and meta-analysis.[9] Combination tablets of metformin and rosiglitazone, and pioglitazone and metformin, are now available.

A previously released glitazone called troglitazone was withdrawn due to cases of fatal hepatotoxicity. Pioglitazone and rosiglitazone have been used extensively and none of the liver toxicity found with troglitazone has been reported. There is therefore now no requirement for 2-monthly liver function test monitoring for glitazones.

Glitazones have been shown to reduce blood pressure slightly, and pioglitazone will reduce total cholesterol by around 15 per cent. It was hoped that these improvements in surrogate markers for cardiovascular disease (CVD) would result in reductions in CVD adverse outcomes. A systematic review[10] of 19 trials has concluded that pioglitazone does reduce the rate of death, myocardial infarction and stroke by 18 per cent compared with controls. However, two similar meta-analyses for rosiglitazone[11,12] suggest an increase in risk of myocardial infarction of around 40 per cent.

Alpha-glucosidase inhibitors (acarbose)

The only agent that is available in the UK is acarbose.

Acarbose reduces the rise in blood glucose seen after a meal by inhibiting the enzyme alpha-glucosidase, which breaks down carbohydrates into monosaccharides in the small intestine. As a result carbohydrates pass further down into the large bowel.

It can reduce HbA_{1c} between 0.6–1 per cent.

It can be used as monotherapy, in any combination with any other agent or agents, and with insulin.

The extra carbohydrate that gets into the large bowel is digested by bowel micro-organisms producing flatulence, bloating and diarrhoea. To try to minimise these side effects the drug should be started at low dose and titrated up. Begin with a 50 mg tablet with one meal each day for 2 weeks, then increase to one 50 mg tablet with each of two meals a day for 2 weeks, then one 50 mg tablet three times daily, increasing to a maximum of 100 mg three times daily. These side effects severely limit its use, and the drug is no longer promoted in the UK.

Incretins

Around 30 years ago it was observed that glucose given orally produced a greater stimulation of insulin release than when an equivalent glucose level was achieved by IV infusion. This was called the 'incretin' effect. It took a number of years before this was explained by the discovery of the gut hormones glucagon-like peptide-1 (GLP-1) and glucose-dependent insulinotropic polypeptide (GIP). These hormones are released by cells in the small bowel in response to food and have a variety of actions, including the stimulation of insulin release from pancreatic beta cells. They are rapidly broken down by the enzyme dipeptidyl peptidase-4 (DPP-4), which is present in the small bowel.

In people with Type 2 diabetes GIP levels are normal in response to a meal but GLP-1 levels are reduced, and so the possibility of using GLP-1 as a therapeutic intervention in diabetes was suggested. GLP-1 has a number of actions that reduce hyperglycaemia, including glucose-dependent stimulation of insulin secretion, glucose-dependent suppression of glucagon secretion, slowing of gastric emptying, improvement in beta cell function, and in animal studies an increase in beta cell mass. GLP-1 has also been associated with reduced food intake and reduction in body weight.

As GLP-1 is broken down so quickly by DPP-4 it would have to be given by continuous intravenous infusion, which makes it impossible to use as a therapy. Huge efforts were therefore made to try to find an entity with GLP-1-like functions but which was resistant to the actions of the DPP-4 enzyme.

Exenatide

This substance is a synthetic version of a protein found in the salivary glands of the Gila monster, a lizard found in the USA. It has the attributes of GLP-1 but is resistant to the action of DPP-4. After an injection, plasma levels are detectable for around 10 hours, making it suitable for twice-daily injection.

In trials exenatide reduces Hb_{A1c} by around 1 per cent as compared with placebo, and there was no difference in Hb_{A1c} reductions between exenatide and insulin glargine or biphasic insulin aspart in open-label non-inferiority studies.[13] Exenatide produces weight loss of around 1.5 kg when compared with placebo and around 5 kg when compared with insulin.[13]

Hypoglycaemia occurs very occasionally when exenatide is used with a sulphonylurea.

The main side effects are dose-dependent nausea and vomiting. It was generally mild to moderate in severity, peaked during the initial 8 weeks of therapy and declined thereafter. Around 4 per cent of patients withdrew from exenatide trials because of adverse GI side effects.

Exenatide is initiated at a dose of 5 mcg twice a day any time within a 60 minute time period before the morning and evening meal. It is increased to a dose of 10 mcg b.d. after 1 month. There is no dose adjustment for meal size or amount of exercise.

It is licensed to be used in combination with metformin and/or a sulphonylurea in patients who have not achieved adequate glycaemic control on maximally tolerated doses of these oral therapies.

The National Institute for Health and Clinical Excellence (NICE) guideline on the management of Type 2 diabetes was published in May 2008.[14]

It suggests that exenatide should only be considered for patients with Type 2 diabetes who have all of the following:

1 ▷ a body mass index over 35 kg/m²
2 ▷ specific problems of a psychological, biochemical or physical nature arising from high body weight
3 ▷ inadequate blood glucose control (Hb_{A1c} above 7.5 per cent) on conventional oral agent therapy after a trial of metformin and sulphonylurea

and

4 ▷ where other high-cost medication such as glitazones or insulin injection therapy would otherwise be started.

DPP-4 inhibitors

Another way of increasing GLP-1 levels in people with Type 2 diabetes would be by inhibiting its breakdown. This can be achieved by using small molecules that can be taken orally. These molecules, termed DPP-4 inhibitors, lower blood glucose and reduce Hb_{A1c} when given orally to people with Type

2 diabetes. Two agents, sitagliptin and vildagliptin, have been launched in the UK and several other DPP-4 inhibitors are in development.

DPP-4 inhibitors lower Hb_{A1c} compared with placebo by 0.74 per cent with similar efficacy as monotherapy or as add-on therapy. Sitagliptin and vild-agliptin have not been compared directly but both appear to lower Hb_{A1c} by a similar amount as compared with placebo. Combining data from four non-inferiority trials, DPP-4 inhibitors were slightly less effective compared with other hypoglycaemic agents (weighted mean difference of 0.21 per cent).[13]

The agents seem weight neutral and in the initial clinical trials appear to be well tolerated, causing no significant adverse events.

Sitagliptin is given as one 100 mg tablet daily. Its initial licence was for it to be used with metformin or a glitazone in people with Type 2 diabetes inadequately controlled by diet, exercise and either metformin or a glita-zone alone. Subsequently it has obtained a licence to be used in triple oral therapy with metformin and sulphonylurea. Vildagliptin is only licensed to be used in dual therapy at present.

Using the current oral agents – initial monotherapy

Metformin is the recommended oral agent for initial monotherapy in people with Type 2 diabetes who are overweight in current national and interna-tional guidelines.[14–17] The reasons for this include that it is well known, it is inexpensive, it does not cause hypoglycaemia, it is weight neutral, and it has been shown to reduce CVD risk in the UKPDS metformin substudy.[4] It should also be considered as oral monotherapy in people who are of normal weight.[15]

The small group of patients who newly present with diabetes who are thin, who eat healthily and who have significant symptoms of hyperglycaemia such as thirst, polydipsia and polyuria are perhaps the only group who may be better treated by a sulphonylurea rather than metformin initially. The sulphonylurea will act more quickly to relieve symptoms. Lack of insulin rather than insulin resistance might be felt to be the major problem in such individuals.

Using the current agents – dual therapy

Once treatment with lifestyle modification followed by metformin therapy is insufficient to optimise glycaemic control, the 2008 NICE guideline[14] recommends the addition of sulphonylurea, as does the IDF guideline.[16]

The reasons for this include the fact that the agents have been around for a long time and are well known, that they act quickly and effectively lower blood glucose, and that they are cheap. The IDF guideline[16] suggests that the addition of a glitazone to metformin for dual therapy could be an option. The ADA/EASD guideline[17] suggests that, after metformin, either a sulphonylurea or a glitazone or insulin initiation might be considered as options for dual therapy. Glitazones have been promoted by their manufacturers for use as second to metformin on the basis that they lower HbA_{1c} as well as sulphonylurea (although they take longer to do this), they do not cause hypoglycaemia, and that they may well lower CVD risk. There is emerging evidence to support the lowering of CVD risk for pioglitazone.[10] The evidence from meta-analysis for rosiglitazone suggests it does not decrease, but rather may increase, risk.[11,12] As glitazones are currently much more expensive than sulphonylurea in the UK it is likely that guidelines in the UK will continue to recommend that for most people sulphonylurea be added to metformin for dual therapy, rather than pioglitazone.

Triple therapy

Once metformin and sulphonylurea taken in dual therapy at maximally tolerated doses are not sufficient for optimal control of glycaemia, what options are available? At present in the UK the options are:

1 ▷ add a glitazone in a 'triple oral therapy' combination
2 ▷ add insulin
3 ▷ add exenatide
4 ▷ add a DPP-4 inhibitor.

There are studies that compare the option of insulin or glitazone in triple therapy.[18,19] The results show similar levels of HbA_{1c} in the group given glitazone in triple oral therapy to the group given basal insulin and dual oral therapy. Depending on how many units of insulin are required the costs of each option can be similar.

In view of the data on glitazones and CVD risk discussed above, pioglitazone at a dose of 30 mg once daily should be the preferred glitazone in the triple oral agent option. When given the choice, a number of patients opt for triple oral therapy rather than two tablets and the injection of insulin.

The only DPP-4 inhibitor licensed to be used in combination with metformin plus sulphonylurea is sitagliptin.

The rapid update of the glycaemic control section of NICE Clinical Guideline 66 was published on 27 May 2009 as Guideline 87.[20] The new recommendations cover DPP-4 inhibitors (sitagliptin, vildagliptin), thiazo-lidinediones (pioglitazone, rosiglitazone), exenatide and insulin.

Guideline 87 continues the recommendation from 66 that lifestyle change alone be used as first treatment. If lifestyle alone does not control glycaemia the guideline recommends metformin monotherapy and, if a second agent is needed, sulphonylurea should be the usual choice. It does say that glitazone or a DPP-4 inhibitor are second-line options to metformin if sulphonylurea is contraindicated or not tolerated. If metformin plus sulphonylurea do not control glycaemia adequately the guideline recommends that a glitazone can be added, or that the DPP-4 inhibitor sitagliptin can be added as it is the DPP-4 inhibitor with a triple-therapy licence. Basal insulin is the recommended third-level choice to be added to metformin plus sulphonylurea, particularly if the person is markedly hyperglycaemic. Exenatide is a third-line option for a patient whose BMI is at or above 35 (for patients of European descent).

Clinical Guideline 87 gives discontinuation recommendations for certain therapies. It says that DPP-4 inhibitors and glitazones should only be continued if there is a 0.5 per cent HB_{A1c} drop in 6 months. It says that exenatide should only be continued if the patient has an HB_{A1c} drop of 1 per cent and a drop of 3 per cent or more of initial body weight in 6 months.

47

Using insulin in those with Type 2 diabetes

When insulin is needed in someone with Type 2 diabetes his or her preference and lifestyle need to be taken into consideration. The most straightforward way to start is to continue metformin and sulphonylurea oral medications and add once-daily basal insulin. Continuing the oral agents when adding insulin reduces the number of units of insulin required, reduces the weight gain associated with insulin therapy, and reduces hypoglycaemia episodes.[21] The long-acting NPH insulins (e.g. insulatard) are the cheapest and so are recommended as the basal insulin of choice in the NICE guideline.[14] They do however cause more hypoglycaemia as compared with the new long-acting insulin analogues, insulin glargine and insulin detemir, and these insulins may be preferred where hypoglycaemia is a concern.

Insulin initiation used to require referral to secondary care but training programmes have been established to enable GPs and practice nurses to acquire these skills and gain experience, so that they can initiate insulin in people with Type 2 diabetes.[22] Patient-initiated up-titration algorithms, usually starting with a dose of basal insulin of 10 units, have been shown to be safe and effective in getting people to an optimal dose of insulin.[23]

Initiating insulin in a person with Type 2 diabetes

1 ▶ Before start of insulin:
  ▷ teach home blood glucose monitoring if not already doing so
  ▷ revise and reinforce dietary principles.

2 ▶ Initiation of insulin:
  ▷ continue on metformin and sulphonylurea oral agents
  ▷ teach insulin injection technique, using injection pen
  ▷ starting dose of 10 units
  ▷ give verbal and written instructions (patient-initiated up-titration algorithm) about increasing insulin dose depending on fasting glucose levels from SMBG
  ▷ teach about hypoglycaemia symptoms and treatment
  ▷ give contact telephone number for advice and help.

3 ▶ Follow-up:
  ▷ by phone after a couple of days and then individualise frequency of calls, depending on progress, need to alter insulin dose and blood glucose control
  ▷ HbA_{1c} every 3 months until stabilised.

Suggested algorithm for glucose-lowering therapies

The following algorithm is based on the NICE 2008 and 2009 guidelines:[14,20]

▷ suboptimal glycaemic control on lifestyle modification – check patient understanding

▷ **BEGIN** metformin 500 mg b.d.

▷ recheck HbA_{1c} at 3 months; if suboptimally controlled **INCREASE** to 1 gm b.d.

▷ (trial metformin MR 1 increasing up to four tablets daily if unable to tolerate generic metformin)

▷ recheck HbA_{1c} after 3 months; if suboptimally controlled **ADD** sulphonyluea, e.g. gliclazide 80 mg b.d.

▷ recheck HbA_{1c} after 3 months; if suboptimally controlled **INCREASE** sulphonylurea (e.g. gliclazide 160 mg b.d.)

▷ recheck HbA_{1c} after 3 months; if suboptimally controlled consider third-line options:

1 ▷ add glitazone
2 ▷ add DPP-4 inhibitor
3 ▷ add exenatide
4 ▷ add basal insulin.

Concordance with therapy

The problem of patients not complying with treatment was first recorded over 2000 years ago when Hippocrates advised the physician 'to be alert to the faults of the patients which make them lie about their taking of the medicines prescribed and when things go wrong, refuse to confess that they have not been taking their medicine'.[24] In a retrospective cohort study from Scotland,[25] 2920 subjects with at least 12 months' prescriptions for oral hypoglycaemic agents were identified, and their adherence to treatment was estimated using data gathered from dispensed prescriptions.

Adequate adherence to treatment, defined as dispensed doses of at least 90 per cent of doses prescribed, was found in only 31 per cent on sulphonylurea monotherapy and 34 per cent on metformin monotherapy. There were significant linear trends of poorer adherence with each increase in daily number of tablets taken, and increase in co-medication.

There are several reasons why people may not take their tablets as prescribed, including:

▷ lack of education or understanding regarding appropriate self-administration and the importance of daily treatment
▷ confusion over which tablets to take when; this may especially occur in older people with developing memory loss
▷ changes in drug or dose regimen
▷ unpleasant side effects
▷ physical problems with opening the packaging or problems reading the label
▷ demands of a busy lifestyle.

We can try to improve concordance with medication by taking some simple, specific actions.

1 ▷ Carefully explain to people what each tablet is for, when it should be taken, and the importance of remembering to take each treatment as prescribed.
2 ▷ Try to minimise the number of tablets to be taken, and the frequency they need to be taken. Once-daily treatments are the ideal from the concordance perspective.
3 ▷ Use treatments that have few if any side effects wherever possible.
4 ▷ Ensure treatments are appropriately packaged and labelling is clear.
5 ▷ Consider pre-filled tablet-dispensing systems if forgetting whether tablets have been taken or not is becoming an issue.

Scenario revisited

David does not want to consider insulin as this would mean he would have to give up his job. He does not want injections, and is not obese so exenatide is not an option he wants to consider.

In discussion he decides to opt for the addition of pioglitazone 30 mg once daily.

After 3 months his Hb_{A1c} has dropped to 7.3 per cent and he feels well. He has put on 2 kg in weight.

After 6 months his Hb_{A1c} has fallen further to 6.9 per cent and his weight has increased by a further 1 kg.

Summary

In relation to the six domains of core or essential competences of being a GP:

1 Primary care management

▷ Understanding of the mechanism of action, efficacy and side effects of diabetes glucose-lowering therapies and how they can be used in monotherapy, dual and triple therapy.
▷ Understanding of the role of insulin in glycaemic lowering in people with Type 2 diabetes.
▷ Understanding the principles and practice of insulin initiation in primary care, dose adjustments and the place of more complex insulin regimes.

2 Person-centred care

▷ To understand the impact of different oral agents on the individual, and the importance of education about their effects to aid concordance.

3 Specific problem-solving

▷ To be able to discuss and assess concordance with therapy.
▷ To be able to help an individual overcome his or her barriers to insulin therapy when insulin is indicated.

4 A comprehensive approach

▷ To be able to discuss and assess glucose-lowering medications in the context of other treatments the individual may need for his or her other co-morbidities.

5 Community orientation

▷ To encourage the individual to get support and help from others with diabetes by attending the local Diabetes UK support group.

6 A holistic approach

▷ To understand the impact any problems with glucose-lowering therapies has on the quality of life of that individual and, in the case of David, his occupation as a bus driver.

References

1 • Diabetes Control and Complications Trial Research Group. The effect of intensive treatment on the development and progression of long term complications in insulin dependent diabetes mellitus *New England Journal of Medicine* 1993; **329**: 977–86.

2 • Nathan D M, Lachin J, Cleary P, *et al*. Diabetes Control and Complications Trial; Epidemiology of Diabetes Interventions and Complications Research Group. Intensive diabetes therapy and carotid intima-media thickness in type 2 diabetes *New England Journal of Medicine* 2003; **348(23)**: 2349–52.

3 • United Kingdom Prospective Diabetes Study Group. Intensive blood glucose control with sulphonylureas or insulin compared with conventional treatment and risk of complications in patients with type 2 diabetes (UKPDS 33) *Lancet* 1998; **352(9131)**; 837–53.

4 • United Kingdom Prospective Diabetes Study Group. Effect of intensive blood glucose control with metformin on complications in overweight patients with type 2 diabetes (UKPDS 34) *Lancet* 1998; **352(9131)**: 854–65.

5 • United Kingdom Prospective Diabetes Study (UKPDS 35). Association of glycaemia with macrovascular and microvascular complications of type 2 diabetes *British Medical Journal* 2000; **321**: 405–11.

6 • Coster S, Guilliford M C, Seed P T, *et al*. Self-monitoring in type 2 diabetes: a meta-analysis *Diabetic Medicine* 2000; **17**: 755–61.

7 • Farmer A, Wade A, Goyder E, *et al*. on behalf of the Diabetes Glycaemic Education and Monitoring Trial Group (DiGEM). Impact of self monitoring of blood glucose in the management of patients with non-insulin treated diabetes: open parallel group randomised trial *British Medical Journal* 2007; **335**: 132–6.

8 • Owens D, Barnett A H, Pickup J, *et al*. Blood glucose self-monitoring in type 1 and type 2 diabetes: reaching a multidisciplinary consensus *Diabetes and Primary Care* 2004; **6**: 8–16.

9 • Largo R M, Singh P P, Nesto R W. Congestive cardiac failure and cardiovascular death in patients with pre-diabetes and type 2 diabetes given thiazolidinediones: a meta-analysis of randomized controlled trials *Lancet* 2007; **370**: 1129–36.

10 • Lincoff A M, Wolski K, Nicholls S J, *et al*. Pioglitazone and risk of cardiovascular events in patients with type 2 diabetes: a meta-analysis of randomized controlled trials *Journal of the American Medical Association* 2007; **298**: 1180–8.

11 • Nissen S E, Wolski K. Effects of rosiglitazone on the risk of myocardial infarction and death from cardiovascular causes *New England Journal of Medicine* 2007; **357**: 2457–71.

12 • Singh S, Loke Y K, Furberg CD. Long-term risk of cardiovascular events with rosiglitazone: a meta-analysis *Journal of the American Medical Association* 2007; **298**: 1189–95.

13 • Amori R E, Lau J, Pittas A G. Efficacy and safety of incretin therapy in type 2 diabetes: systematic review and meta-analysis *Journal of the American Medical Association* 2007; **298**: 194–206.

14 • National Institute for Health and Clinical Excellence. *Clinical Guideline 66, Type 2 Diabetes: national clinical guideline for management in primary and secondary care* London: NICE, 2008.

15 • National Institute for Health and Clinical Excellence. *Management of Type 2 diabetes: management of blood glucose* London: NICE, 2002.

16 • International Diabetes Foundation. *Global Guideline for Type 2 Diabetes* Brussels: IDF, 2005, www.idf.org/home/index.cfm?node=1457 [accessed July 2009].

17 • Nathan D M, Buse J B, Davidson M B, *et al*. Management of hyperglycaemia in type 2 diabetes: a consensus algorithm for the initiation and adjustment of therapy. A consensus statement from the American Diabetes Association and the European Association for the Study of Diabetes *Diabetes Care* 2006; **29**: 1963–72.

18 • Aljabri K, Kosak S, Thompson D M. Addition of pioglitazone or bedtime insulin to maximal doses of sulphonylurea and metformin in type 2 diabetes patients with poor glucose control: a prospective randomized study *American Journal of Medicine* 2004; **116**: 230–5.

19 • Rosenstock J, Sugimoto D, Strange P, *et al*. Triple therapy in type 2 diabetes *Diabetes Care* 2006; **29**: 554–9.

20 • National Institute for Health and Clinical Excellence. *Clinical Guideline 87, Type 2 Diabetes: newer agents* London: NICE, 2009.

21 • Gadsby R. Using insulin earlier in the treatment of type 2 diabetes *British Journal of Diabetes and Vascular Disease* 2003; **3**: 119–22.

22 • Warwick Medical School. *Diabetes Care and Management* www2.warwick.ac.uk/fac/med/research/themes/diabetes/ [accessed July 2009].

23 • Davies M, Storms F, Shutler S, *et al*. ATLANTUS Study Group. Improvement of glycemic control in subjects with poorly controlled type 2 diabetes: comparison of two treatment algorithms using insulin glargine *Diabetes Care* 2005; **28**: 1282–8.

24 • Sawyer S. *Adherence: whose responsibility?* www.nationalasthma.org.au/html/strategy/cam/cam006.asp [accessed July 2009].

25 • Donnan P T, MacDonald T M, Morris A D for the DARTS/MEMO Collaboration. Adherence to prescribed oral hypoglycaemic medication in a population of patients with Type 2 diabetes: a retrospective cohort study *Diabetic Medicine* 2002; **19**: 279–84.

Macrovascular complications in diabetes mellitus

5

Scenario

Tom is a 57-year-old man who has had Type 2 diabetes for 12 years and hypertension for 14 years. His current medications are metformin 500 mg two tablets b.d., gliclazide 80 mg two tablets b.d., simvastatin 40 mg daily, and lisinopril 20 mg daily. He last attended the diabetes clinic 6 weeks ago when his Hb$_{A1c}$ was 7.1 per cent; his total cholesterol was 4.9 mmol/l and blood pressure 140/80. He has no microalbuminuria and his estimated glomerular filtration rate (eGFR) is 64.

He presents with a 4-week history of tightness in his chest on exercise.

▶ *How would you manage his chest tightness and what changes might you make to his coronary heart disease (CHD) prevention regime?*

The risk

The macrovascular complications of diabetes include myocardial infarction, stroke and peripheral vascular disease. The risks of macrovascular disease are significantly raised in people with diabetes. Cardiovascular risk is increased two- to four-fold in Type 2 diabetes. Up to 75 per cent of people with Type 2 diabetes will die of cardiovascular disease, and life expectancy is reduced by around 10 years by Type 2 diabetes.[1]

In some research studies, a patient with Type 2 diabetes has been found to be as much at risk of having a myocardial infarction as someone who does not have diabetes but has already had a myocardial infarction. Several studies have investigated this idea in different populations and study settings. Five have supported the idea of risk equivalence, while eight have contradicted it.[2] This variation in risk is explained in a more recent paper, which used a population of 4549 Native Americans with a high prevalence of diabetes. It looked at the influence of single and multiple risk factors on the 10-year cumulative incidence of fatal and non-fatal CHD in diabetic and non-diabetic men and women, with and without baseline cardiovascular disease (CVD). They found the CVD risk in people with diabetes depended on whether they had concomitant risk factors such as microalbuminuria, hypertension, smoking status, low HDL cholesterol and raised triglycerides. Most individuals had only one or two risk factors, and had a 10-year cumulative incidence of CHD of less than 20 per cent. However, those with multiple risk factors had a 10-year cumulative incidence of over 40 per cent, equivalent to that of people with a previous infarction.[2] So whether a study finds risk equivalence or not will depend on the risk factor profiles of the individuals making up that population.

Reducing risk

For patients with Type 2 diabetes without known cardiovascular disease, there is good trial evidence that good control of blood pressure, glycaemia and treatment with a statin that lowers cholesterol can reduce risk. There is limited evidence from the Steno-2 study that combining all these interventions can give greater risk reductions than any one of the individual interventions.[3] The Steno-2 study was an open parallel trial of 160 patients with Type 2 diabetes and microalbuminuria. Eighty had conventional treatment in accordance with national guidelines from their GPs, with referral as necessary. Eighty had intensive treatment with stepwise implementation of behaviour modification and drug therapy that targeted hyperglycaemia (HbA_{1c} below 6.5 per cent), hypertension (BP below 130/80), and dyslipidaemia (triglycerides below 1.7, cholesterol below 4.5). All patients in both groups were given aspirin and an angiotensin-converting enzyme (ACE) inhibitor.

The intensive group were also given vitamins E and C, and folic acid. After a mean follow-up of 7.8 years one or more cardiovascular events (death from cardiovascular causes, non-fatal stroke or myocardial infarct, coronary or peripheral revascularisation or amputation as a result of ischaemia) had occurred in 44 per cent in the conventional group but in only 24 per cent in the intensive group. The authors calculate that 5 patients need to be treated for 7.8 years to prevent one cardiovascular event.

Many of the clinical indicator targets in the Quality and Outcomes Framework (QoF) are designed to ensure that people with Type 2 diabetes have their CVD risk factors measured and managed to ensure that CVD risk is reduced.

Good blood pressure control to reduce CVD risk

The United Kingdom Prospective Diabetes Study (UKPDS) began as a study of glycaemic control in people newly diagnosed with Type 2 diabetes. It then had a blood pressure control study embedded into it.

In the blood pressure study 1148 people with hypertension and Type 2 diabetes were randomised to a tight control arm or a less tight control arm. The final mean difference between the two groups was 10/5 mmHg (144/82 in the tight control group as against 154/87 in the other group). Over 9 years those in the tight control group had significant reductions in morbidity and mortality, with:

▷ 32 per cent reduction in diabetes-related death
▷ 44 per cent reduction in fatal and non-fatal stroke
▷ 56 per cent reduction in congestive cardiac failure
▷ 37 per cent reduction in developing microvascular complications.

The tightly controlled were treated with the beta blocker atenolol or the ACE inhibitor captopril, but the study was not sufficiently powered statistically to say which agent was superior.[4]

The Hypertension Optimal Treatment Trial (HOT) randomised 18,790 patients with hypertension into three groups aiming to achieve diastolic pressures of below 90, below 85 and below 80 in each group. The trial contained about 1500 patients with Type 2 diabetes. There were significant reductions in cardiovascular morbidity and mortality in the tightest controlled group, with a relative risk reduction of 50 per cent.[5]

QoF goals for lowering blood pressure

There are two clinical indicators specifically relating to blood pressure. One is a process indicator for blood pressure recording (DM11) and the other a quality indicator for blood pressure below 145/85 (DM12):

▷ DM11 is the percentage of patients with diabetes who have a record of the blood pressure in the last 15 months; minimum threshold = 40 per cent; maximum threshold to earn full 3 available points = 90 per cent
▷ DM12 is the percentage of patients with diabetes in whom the blood pressure is 145/85 or less; minimum threshold = 40 per cent; maximum threshold to gain the full 18 available points = 60 per cent.

Most guidelines, e.g. the new National Service Framework (NSF) guidelines, recommend a target level below 140/80, and recommend a target of

55

below 130/80 if there is evidence of eye, kidney or cerebrovascular damage.[6]

Recommended treatments to lower blood pressure

Most guidelines recommend an ACE inhibitor, as it can effectively lower blood pressure and offers some degree of renal protection. Cough is a common side effect of ACE inhibitor therapy and if cough means that ACE inhibitor is not tolerated then an angiotensin receptor blocker (ARB) should be used. Patients of Afro-Caribbean descent may not respond well to ACE inhibitor therapy, and in this group a calcium channel blocker may be the best first-line blood pressure-lowering therapy.

If a second agent is required, a calcium channel blocker or a thiazide may be added. Both can be used if three agents are needed. If a fourth agent is needed an alpha blocker or a beta blocker can be added, or both if a fifth agent is needed.

Prescribing a statin to reduce CVD risk

There is good trial data to recommend the use of statin therapy to reduce CVD risk in patients with diabetes.

The Heart Protection Study (HPS)[7] examined data from 5963 patients with diabetes (29 per cent of all patients studied) and demonstrated that the incidence of major vascular events in these patients was reduced by 20 per cent with simvastatin 40 mg compared with placebo; this reduction was similar to that observed for the entire study population. This study enrolled people with total cholesterol levels above 3.5 mmol/l. The results of the HPS suggest that it is statin treatment, rather than reduction of cholesterol to any specific, arbitrary figure, that produces the benefit.

The Collaborative Atorvastatin Diabetes Study (CARDS) study looked at 2838 people with Type 2 diabetes and randomised them to atorvastatin 10 mg or placebo. The risk reduction for a CHD event was reduced by 37 per cent.[8]

All the statin studies published so far suggest that people with diabetes gain at least as much benefit from statin therapy as people without diabetes. However, because the relative risk of CHD is two- to four-fold higher, the absolute benefit of statin therapy is likely to be greater.

Statin treatment and cholesterol targets for people with Type 2 diabetes

As simvastatin 40 mg once daily has come off patent, it is now cheap at around £2 to £3 per month and is therefore very cost-effective. It also has an evidence base from the HPS study. It is recommended[6] that it be given to all people with Type 2 diabetes over the age of 40 years unless CVD risk seems unusually low.

Intensification of cholesterol-lowering therapy using a more effective statin or adding ezetimibe (an agent that blocks cholesterol absorption) should be considered for patients with Type 2 diabetes who have not had a myocardial infarction but who are assessed as having a very high CVD risk (those with microalbuminuria, proteinuria, chronic kidney disease or other severe risk factor profile).[6] In these patients the target for total cholesterol should be 4 mmol/l or below with an LDL cholesterol of 2 mmol/l or below, in line with patients who have already had a myocardial infarction.

57

QoF and CHD risk reduction targeting cholesterol

There is a process indicator for cholesterol recording (DM16) and a quality indicator for cholesterol below 5 mmol/l (DM17):

▷ DM16 is the percentage of patients with diabetes who have a record of total cholesterol in the previous 15 months; minimum threshold = 40 per cent; maximum threshold to earn full available 3 points = 90 per cent
▷ DM 17 is the percentage of patients with diabetes whose last measured total cholesterol within previous 15 months is 5 or less; minimum threshold = 40 per cent; maximum threshold to earn full available 3 points = 70 per cent.

Good glycaemic control to reduce CVD risk

This is covered in Chapter 4.

Giving aspirin to reduce CVD risk

The evidence for the benefit of giving aspirin comes from populations who have already had a coronary event, i.e. secondary prevention. Two trials of the use of aspirin in primary prevention in people with diabetes showed non-statistically significant results.

Most guidelines however suggest the use of low-dose aspirin 75 mg daily in patients with diabetes for primary prevention, provided they have controlled blood pressure (less than 145/90) and are above 50 years of age.[6] It is recommended that aspirin 75 mg daily be considered for all people with diabetes who have evidence of cardiovascular disease.

Scenario revisited

On further questioning the chest tightness appears to be due to new-onset angina. An ECG performed in the surgery is normal. After discussion with Tom you decide to refer him to a cardiologist who arranges a treadmill stress test. This is positive and so Tom is referred for coronary angiography.

As CHD has now been diagnosed after discussion with Tom he agrees to take aspirin 75 mg once daily. As simvastatin 40 mg daily is not reducing Tom's total cholesterol to the target of below 4.0 mmol/l that the NICE guideline[6] suggests, there are three possible courses of action:

1 ▷ increase to simvastatin 80 mg (two of 40 mg)
2 ▷ change to a more potent statin
3 ▷ add ezetimibe to 40 mg simvastatin.

In consultation with Tom you decide to change to the more potent statin, atorvastatin 20 mg once daily, with a plan to increase to 40 mg if required to achieve the target.

Summary

In relation to the six domains of core or essential competences of being a GP:

---

1 Primary care management

▷ Identifying the level of CHD risk in people with Type 2 diabetes and prescribing appropriate therapies for primary prevention.
▷ Titrating lipid-lowering and blood pressure-lowering therapies to achieve appropriate targets in primary prevention.
▷ Recording data to enable QoF targets to be obtained.

2 Person-centred care

▷ Discussion and negotiation to determine the level of risk for that individual and to agree targets for prevention.

3 Specific problem-solving skills

▷ Understanding the level of CHD risk for any given individual.

4 A comprehensive approach

▷ Discussion with the individual to determine his or her level of understanding of CHD risk in the context of co-morbidities and age, and his or her desire for medication to reduce the risk.

5 Community orientation

▷ Recall programme in GP practice in order to screen for new patients with diabetes and to follow up those diagnosed for an annual review.

6 A holistic approach

▷ Discussing with the individual how important to him or her primary prevention is in the context of his or her life and co-morbidities.

References

1 • Donnelly R, Emslie-Smith AM, Gardner ID, *et al*. ABC of arterial & venous disease: vascular complications of diabetes *British Medical Journal* 2000; **320**: 1062–6.

2 • Howard B V, Best L G, Galloway J M, *et al*. Coronary heart disease in diabetes depends on concomitant risk factors *Diabetes Care* 2006; **29**: 391–7.

3 • Gaede P, Vedel P, Larson N, *et al*. Multifactorial intervention and cardiovascular disease in patients with type 2 diabetes *New England Journal of Medicine* 2003; **348**: 383–93.

4 • UKPDS Group. Tight blood pressure control and risk of macrovascular and microvascular complications in type 2 diabetes (UKPDS 38) *British Medical Journal* 1998; **317**: 703–13.

5 • Hansson L, Zanchetti A, Carruthers S G, *et al*. Effects of intensive blood pressure lowering and low dose aspirin therapy in patients with hypertension: principal results of the Hypertension Optimal Treatment (HOT) randomised trial *Lancet* 1998; **351**: 1755–62.

6 • National Institute for Health and Clinical Excellence. *Clinical Guideline 66, Type 2 Diabetes: the management of type 2 diabetes* London: NICE, 2008, www.nice.org.uk/nicemedia/pdf/CG66NICEGuideline.pdf [accessed July 2009].

7 • Heart Protection Study Group. MRC/BHF Heart Protection Study of cholesterol lowering with simvastatin in 20,536 high-risk individuals: a randomised placebo-controlled trial *Lancet* 2002; **360**: 7–22.

8 • Colhoun H M, Betteridge D J, Durrington P N, *et al.* Prevention of cardiovascular disease with atorvastatin in type 2 diabetes: the CARDS multicentre randomized, placebo controlled trial *Lancet* 2004; **364**: 685–96.

Microvascular complications in diabetes mellitus

6

Scenario

Michael is 38 years old and has had Type 1 diabetes for 28 years. He is married with two children aged 11 and 8, and works in a printing company where he spends a lot of the day looking at a computer screen.

His blood pressure is 130/80 and two urine tests have confirmed microalbuminuria. He is on a basal bolus insulin regime, but no other medications, and is not doing any self-monitoring of his blood glucose at present. His recent HbA1c was 7.8 per cent. Michael's body mass index (BMI) is 23.5 kg/m² he goes to the gym three times a week and feels that he is keeping fit.

He has defaulted from his last three diabetes clinic appointments at the hospital because he says that he cannot afford to take time off work. He attends the practice diabetes clinic as he can get an appointment after work.

At his last screening he was found to have background diabetic retinopathy, and he comes to ask if he is likely to develop problems with his eyesight as a result. He is worried because he says he needs good vision to do his job.

▶ *How would you answer his concerns about his eyes?*

Introduction

The microvascular complications of diabetes are:

▷ nephropathy
▷ retinopathy
▷ neuropathy.

They tend to occur together so that if a person with diabetes has no signs of retinopathy, but has signs of nephropathy, a non-diabetes cause of the nephropathy needs to be considered.

Erectile dysfunction will also be discussed in this chapter.

There is strong evidence that good blood glucose control with an HbA1c of 7 per cent reduces microvascular complications, in both Type 1 diabetes (with evidence from the DCCT study) and in Type 2 diabetes (with evidence from the UKPDS study). (See Chapter 4 for a discussion of the evidence for these two studies.) Strategies other than good blood glucose control will therefore be discussed in this chapter.

Preventing nephropathy

Not everyone with diabetes will develop nephropathy, but in those that do a progressive natural history has been described. This is best documented in Type 1 diabetes.

In the first few years of living with diabetes, kidney function is normal and there is variable excretion of only tiny amounts of protein, less than 30 mg in 24 hours.

Later, often after 8 to 10 years of living with Type 1 diabetes, microalbuminuria may develop. This stage may last for 10 years. People at this stage often have a normal blood pressure.

After about 20 plus years of living with Type 1 diabetes, frank proteinuria may develop. This continues on with progressive renal impairment, a rising serum creatinine level and hypertension. It leads to the need for renal replacement therapy (dialysis or transplantation) after around 25 to 30 years of living with diabetes.

The cumulative incidence of microalbuminuria in patients with Type 1 diabetes for 30 years is around 40 per cent.[1] Around 20 per cent of people with Type 1 diabetes develop proteinuria after 25 years of living with diabetes.[2]

ACE inhibitors, when given to people with Type 1 diabetes who are normotensive but who have microalbuminuria, can delay or postpone the progression of nephropathy.[3] Most published studies of ACE therapy showing these benefits have been at the higher end of their therapeutic dose ranges.

In Type 2 diabetes most people with microalbuminuria also have hypertension. The presence of microalbuminuria is a marker for increased cardiovascular risk, and a number of people with microalbuminuria will die of coronary heart disease (CHD) before they have time to develop end-stage renal disease.

Treatment with an ACE inhibitor is also beneficial. One study looked at the ACE inhibitor ramipril in people with Type 2 diabetes for a mean of 4.5 years. The drug reduced cardiovascular mortality by 25 per cent in people with normal serum creatinine levels and in those with mild renal insufficiency.[4]

Several studies have also shown the benefit of angiotensin 2 antagonists (AT2s). In one study 5 per cent of microalbuminuric Type 2 patients developed diabetic nephropathy when treated with irbesartan compared with 15 per cent in a control group over 2 years. This effect was independent of blood pressure.[5] At the stage of diabetic nephropathy with a reduced glomerular filtration rate, 17 per cent of Type 2 patients treated with irbesartan doubled their serum creatinine level over 2.6 years as against 25 per cent in a control group.[6]

Measuring microalbuminuria

Microalbuminuria can occur in healthy people after they have been standing for a while; this is why tests are done after a period of recumbency. An early-morning specimen is used, as for most people this is after sleep. Microalbuminuria can occur after exercise or during a febrile illness, and so testing should be delayed if these are present.

Near-patient testing strips are available to be used to detect microalbuminuria, but their cost, and the fact that they do not give a figure for the albumin:creatinine ratio (A:C ratio), has meant that they are not widely used.

Microalbuminuria is usually detected by sending an early-morning urine sample to a laboratory for the detection of the A:C ratio. A ratio greater than 2.5 mg/mmol for men and 3.5 for women indicates microalbuminuria.

If the A:C ratio is normal the patient can be left for a repeat check in one year. However, If the stick test or the A:C ratio is abnormal the NICE guideline states that they need to be repeated twice within a month and if two out of three tests are positive microalbuminuria is said to be present.

There are Quality and Outcomes Framework (QoF) targets for measuring microalbuminuria and ensuring that patients with diabetes and microalbuminuria are treated with an ACE or AT2 drug. The other measure of renal function with a QoF target is the measurement of serum creatinine. Laboratories in the UK are now combining this blood result with the patient's age and sex to report an estimated glomerular filtration rate (eGFR). Serum creatinine alone may give an inaccurate picture of renal function. It is possible to have a fairly normal serum creatinine but to have significantly reduced renal function. The new measure of eGFR brings some added precision to the measurement of renal function. eGFR is used to classify chronic kidney disease (CKD) into five stages (see Table 6.1).

Table 6.1 ○ *eGFR and the stages of CKD*

eGFR	Stage
At or above 90	CKD stage 1
60–89	CKD stage 2
30–59	CKD stage 3
15–29	CKD stage 4
Below 15	CKD stage 5

If there is no proteinuria or haematuria then CKD stages 1 and 2 are normal. Referral to nephrology services should normally be made for people with stages 4 and 5, unless the patient is elderly and there is evidence that his or her eGFR is stable.

Preventing blindness by reducing retinopathy

Diabetic retinopathy is the leading cause of blindness in the UK in people of working age. Many people who have diabetic retinopathy will be asymptomatic and have good vision. Even people with sight-threatening retinopathy may be asymptomatic.

There is convincing evidence that regular surveillance for diabetic retinopathy in people with diabetes, and early laser treatment of those identified as having sight-threatening retinopathy, can reduce the incidence of new visual impairment and blindness.[7,8]

The key issue is therefore to identify those people with sight-threatening retinopathy who will benefit from prophylactic treatment to prevent visual loss. This is being implemented in the UK through a retinal screening programme based on digital retinal photography through dilated pupils. At present screening is every year and there is a QoF target for retinal screening.

A call and recall system has to be set in place to ensure that people are invited to attend for retinal screening on a yearly basis. This is usually arranged as part of the retinal screening programme. There are several models to deliver retinal screening occurring across the UK. In one the screening may take place in the community, often on the practice premises, when the mobile retinal screening team with the camera visits the practice. In another the patient to be screened visits a centre where there is a static camera; these are often sited at a diabetes centre at a hospital. A third model is to use optometrists who have digital cameras on their premises to photograph the retina.

Patients need to be made aware that their pupils will be dilated for the screening photograph and they should not therefore drive for about 4 hours or so afterwards.

Information leaflets have been written to give to patients to explain about the screening process, the process of laser treatment if required, and giving advice about being accompanied to the screening appointment.[9]

If the photograph shows no retinopathy, further screening will take place on a yearly basis. However, if retinopathy is found, the extent of the retinopathy will be assessed. If it is felt that laser therapy is indicated then rapid referral to an ophthalmology department is arranged for this treatment. If retinopathy is detected but it is not of sufficient severity to require immediate laser therapy, the patient will be recalled for further observation within the screening programme.

Preventing amputations by stopping foot ulceration

Foot problems in diabetes result from neuropathy, which leads to loss of protective pain sensation in the feet and from ischaemia due to peripheral vascular disease.

Between 20 and 40 per cent of people with diabetes are estimated to have neuropathy depending on how it is defined and measured, and about 5 per cent have a foot ulcer.[10] Foot ulcers that get infected may lead to amputation. The incidence rate of diabetes-related lower-limb amputation in one community study in the Tayside area of Scotland was 248 per 100,000 person years, which was 12.4 times higher than for the general population.[11]

Diabetic peripheral neuropathy is usually asymptomatic, and the gradual loss of protective pain sensation usually is not perceived by the person as it develops. Thus there are people with diabetes who have risk factors for foot ulceration and amputation of which they are not aware.

Approximately 50 per cent of people with diabetes who attend dedicated foot clinics just have neuropathy. The other 50 per cent have neuropathy plus some degree of reduced blood flow resulting from generalised atherosclerosis that produces tissue ischaemia in the foot.[12] Pure ischaemia without neuropathy is rare. Poor glycaemic control, duration of diabetes, and adverse socioeconomic conditions are other factors associated with increased risk of foot ulceration.

Feet that are at risk due to neuropathy or ischaemia do not spontaneously ulcerate. Minor trauma is usually the additional factor that precipitates ulceration. The patient with loss of protective pain sensation due to neuropathy may get trauma through thermal damage (e.g. walking on hot sand on holiday), chemical damage (e.g. use of corn cures) or through mechanical trauma (e.g. tightly fitting shoes, standing on a stone or a drawing pin).

Foot ulcers are susceptible to infection, which may spread rapidly, causing overwhelming tissue destruction. This process is the main reason for amputation in people with diabetes who have neuropathy. The pathway to amputation is thus a foot at risk, minor trauma, ulceration, spreading infection and amputation.

Strategies to reduce the risk of amputation include:

▷ early recognition of the at-risk foot by annual screening
▷ prompt referral for assessment of risk, with intensive education and regular follow up for people who have 'foot at risk' detected
▷ rapid referral for intensive treatment of foot ulcers in multidisciplinary foot clinics.[10, 11]

Screening for feet at risk

There are two clinical indicators in the QoF framework for annual screening for 'foot at risk'. These are the palpation of the dorsalis pedis and posterior tibial foot pulses and the detection of neuropathy in the foot.

The pulses can be easily palpated using the fingers.

The NICE guideline [10] states that there is a good evidence base for the use of the 10 g nylon monofilament to detect neuropathy. The monofilament is easy to use, light and cheap.[13]

The filament is applied to at least five sites on the foot (but not over callus, which is an area of dry, hard and often fissured skin) until it buckles, which occurs at 10 g of linear pressure when the patient is asked to detect its presence. If it cannot be felt, protective pain sensation is lost and neuropathy is present.

Diabetic neuropathy usually begins peripherally, so that if the patient can feel the monofilament on the toes, he or she does not usually have neuropathy. Isolated areas of apparent insensitivity in other parts of the foot are of less significance.

Referral of someone with a foot at risk

If someone is detected at screening as having a foot at risk through the absence of foot pulses or the inability to detect the 10 g nylon monofilament he or she needs to be referred straight away to the community 'foot at risk' clinic. Here podiatrists will further assess the degree of risk, provide extra education, and give advice about footwear. They will then follow up every few months depending on the degree of risk.

Referral of someone with a foot ulcer

If someone develops a foot ulcer they need prompt referral to a multidisciplinary foot service for treatment of infection, stabilisation of blood glucose, debridement and offloading of the ulcer, and appropriate dressings.

Erectile dysfunction

Erectile dysfunction (ED) is the major sexual problem affecting men with diabetes. It occurs in 30 per cent of all men who have diabetes and 55 per cent of those over 60 years of age.[14] The prevalence and impact of erectile failure in diabetes is probably underestimated because of medical and social taboos.

Its aetiology is multifactorial. The main two factors are:

▷ atheroma causing reduced microvascular blood flow to the penis
▷ damage to the autonomic nervous system.

Psychological factors may also play a part in some people.

Infections, e.g. balanitis, are common in men with poorly controlled diabetes and can cause malaise, local pain and anxiety, which may all contribute to worsening ED. Some diabetes drugs, such as beta blockers and thiazide diuretics used to treat hypertension, some antidepressants and some anxiolytic agents, are also associated with ED. Alcohol in excess may also cause ED.

Now that people know that an oral therapy is available to treat ED, men with diabetes are becoming more willing to discuss this microvascular complication. The emergence of oral agents that suppress the enzyme phosphodiesterase type 5 (PDE5) has been a very important breakthrough in the treatment of ED. They suppress PDE5, which occurs naturally in the erectile tissue of the penis. PDE5 breaks down intracellular guanosine monophosphate (cGMP), which is produced during arousal and causes the vascular changes that lead to erection of the penis.

Sildenafil is taken an hour or so before intended intercourse. It does not by itself produce arousal, but allows an erection to occur during sexual foreplay. It is available in 25, 50 or 100 mg tablets. The stronger doses are needed in people with diabetes and an up to 60 per cent response rate has been reported.[14]

Two other PDE5 inhibitors have also been launched in the UK. One is tadalafil and the other vardenafil. These agents also seem to be effective in people with diabetes. It would also be interesting to carry out studies that compare the effectiveness of the three PDE5s with each other, in people with diabetes.

PDE5 inhibitors can interact with nitrate-containing medications to cause hypotension. Therefore they should not be used in people with ischaemic heart disease who are taking nitrate therapy.

Vacuum tumescence devices consist of cylinders into which the penis is placed, and from which air is removed creating a vacuum, which then produces an erection. They can be very effective and are free of systemic side effects. Few large-scale studies have been reported so success rates in diabetes are difficult to ascertain. It is a treatment option for people with diabetes who are not helped by oral PDE5 inhibitors or people on nitrate therapy in whom they are contraindicated.

Discussing erectile dysfunction

It is a difficult subject for the person with diabetes and the healthcare professional to bring up in the consultation. Questions like 'A number of men with diabetes get problems with getting an erection. Is this a problem that is bothering you?' can introduce the subject into the consultation in a relatively non-threatening way.

ED due to a complication of diabetes needs to be distinguished from psychological causes of ED, and a brief history about the ED needs to be taken. The following table lists factors in the history that may help to distinguish them.

Table 6.2 ○ **Psychological and microvascular causes of erectile dysfunction**

	Psychological	Microvascular
Onset	Often sudden	Gradual
Permanence	Intermittent or partial	Total
Nocturnal erections	Sometimes	Never
Psychological symptoms	Present	Absent
Other microvascular complications	Often absent	Present
Erection lost on penetration	Often happens	No erections

Treatment options

Psychological causes of ED may improve after discussion and counselling. For ED caused by diabetes, the treatment options of intra-urethral alprostadil, penile alprostadil by injection, vacuum devices and oral PDE5 inhibitors can be discussed.

In my experience most opt for a trial of oral therapy with a PDE5 inhibitor. Doses at the upper end of the dose range are usually needed. Diabetes is one of the conditions that allows four oral tablets of a PDE5 inhibitor a month to be prescribed free on the NHS.

Scenario revisited

After a long discussion with Michael you agree together to arrange a late-afternoon appointment at the hospital diabetes clinic to discuss increasing his insulin doses. It is necessary to get his Hb_{A1c} nearer to 7 per cent in order to reduce the risk of progression of his microvascular complications of nephropathy (as evidenced by his microalbuminuria) and his retinopathy. You are able to reassure him that his retinopathy is only background at present and as such will not affect his vision.

He agrees to begin the ACE inhibitor lisinopril at a starting dose of 2.5 mg daily, with an aim to titrate up the dose to 20 mg over the next 8 weeks, providing this is tolerated. You reassure him that the chances of hypotension are small and that there is good evidence that this, along with good blood glucose control, will reduce the chances of progression of his microvascular disease.

In view of the microalbuminuria he is at increased risk of CHD and he agrees to take simvastatin 40 mg daily in primary prevention. Simvastatin 40 mg once daily is recommended as the initial statin therapy of choice in the NICE Type 2 guidelines.[15]

His foot examination is normal. You enquire whether he has any concerns about erectile dysfunction and he says things are okay.

Summary

In relation to the six domains of core or essential competences of being a GP:

---

1 Primary care management

▷ Recognition of the signs and symptoms of the microvascular complications of diabetes and their management in primary care as part of the annual review.
▷ Referral of people found to have 'at risk' feet for further evaluation, education and follow-up to the 'foot at risk' clinic.

2 Person-centred care

▷ To understand the impact of microvascular complications on the individual and his or her concerns.
▷ To be able to discuss the issue of erectile dysfunction and whether this is a concern to the individual.

3 Specific problem-solving skills

▷ To be able to discuss and negotiate a return to the hospital clinic to review glycaemic control as appropriate.
▷ Relating microalbuminuria and eGFR measurements.
▷ Discussion with the local consultant diabetologist and diabetes specialist nurse (DSN) to get an appointment at the hospital clinic as soon as possible.

4 A comprehensive approach

▷ To understand that the microvascular complications of diabetes often occur together and therefore, if a person has one detected, enquiry and investigation need to take place to check for the others.
▷ To ensure that all individuals with diabetes registered at the practice receive a comprehensive annual review examination.

5 Community orientation

▷ To ensure that all people registered at the practice receive an annual retinal screening examination to national standards.

6 A holistic approach

▷ To understand the impact any microvascular complications are having on the patients and their lives.
▷ Enquiring about and providing treatment for individuals with ED.

References

1 • Parving HH, Hommel E, Mathiesen E, *et al*. Prevalence of microalbuminuria, arterial hypertension, retinopathy and neuropathy in patients with insulin dependent diabetes mellitus *British Medical Journal* 1988; **296**; 156–60.

2 • Stephenson J, Fuller JH, the EURODIAB IDDM Complications Study Group. Microvascular and acute complications in IDDM patients: the EURODIAB IDDM Complications Study *Diabetologia* 1994; **37(3)**: 278–85.

3 • Mathiesen E, Hommel E, Giesel J, *et al*. Efficacy of captopril in postponing nephropathy in normotensive insulin dependent diabetic patients with microalbuminuria *British Medical Journal* 1991; **303**: 81–7.

4 • Heart Outcomes Prevention Evaluation Study Investigators. Effects of ramipril on cardiovascular and microvascular outcomes in people with diabetes mellitus: results of the HOPE study and MICROHOPE substudy *Lancet* 2000; **355**: 253–9.

5 • Parving HH, Lehnert H, Brocher-Mortensen J, *et al*. The effect of irbesartan on the development of diabetic nephropathy in patients with type 2 diabetes *New England Journal of Medicine* 2001; **345**: 870–8.

6 • Lewis EJ, Hunsicker LG, Clarke WR, *et al*. Renoprotective effect of the angiotensin-receptor antagonist irbesartan in patients with nephropathy due to type 2 diabetes *New England Journal of Medicine* 2001; **345**: 851–60.

7 • Klein R, Klein BEK, Moss SE, *et al*. The Wisconsin Epidemiological Study of Diabetic Retinopathy 111: prevalence and risk of diabetic retinopathy when age at diagnosis is 30 years or more *Archives of Ophthalmology* 1984; **102**: 527–32.

8 • Ferris F. Early photocoagulation in patients with either type 1 or type 2 diabetes *Transactions of the American Ophthalmological Society* 1996; **94**: 505–37.

9 • www.retinalscreening.nhs.uk/pages/ [accessed July 2009].

10 • National Institute for Health and Clinical Excellence. *Clinical Guideline 10, Type 2 Diabetes: prevention and management of foot problems* London: NICE, 2004, www.nice.org.uk/nicemedia/pdf/CG010NICEguideline.pdf [accessed July 2009].

11 • Morris AD, McAlpine R, Steinke D, *et al*. Diabetes and lower limb amputations in the community: a retrospective cohort study. DARTS/MEMO Collaboration *Diabetes Care* 1998; **21**: 738–41.

12 • Gadsby R, McInnes A. The at-risk foot: the role of the primary care team in achieving St Vincent targets for reducing amputation *Diabetic Medicine* 1998; **15(Suppl 3)**: S61–4.

13 • Kumar S, Fernando DJS, Veves A, *et al*. Semmes–Weinstein monofilaments: a simple, effective and inexpensive screening device for identifying diabetic patients at risk of foot ulceration *Diabetes Research and Clinical Practice* 1991; **13**: 63–8.

14 • Rendell MS, Rajfer J, Wicker P, *et al*. for the Sildenafil Diabetes Study Group. Sildenafil for treatment of erectile dysfunction in men with diabetes: a randomised controlled study *Journal of the American Medical Association* 1999; **281**: 421–6.

15 • National Institute for Health and Clinical Excellence. *Clinical Guideline 66, Type 2 Diabetes: the management of type 2 diabetes* London: NICE, 2008, www.nice.org.uk/nicemedia/pdf/CG66NICEGuideline.pdf [accessed July 2009].

Ethnic, cultural and psycho-social aspects of diabetes

7

Scenario

Jaswinder is a 43-year-old woman of South Asian ethnicity who has had Type 2 diabetes for 5 years. She is obese with a body mass index (BMI) of 31. She is on metformin 500 mg two b.d., gliclazide 80 mg b.d. and simvastatin 40 mg daily. Her blood pressure is 130/80 on no medication, and her total cholesterol is 4.2 mmol/l. Her latest Hb_{A1c} is 9.7 per cent, up from 7.2 per cent 6 months ago.

She has four children aged between 7 and 17 years. She doesn't speak much English.

She attends the surgery for a diabetes review with her 17-year-old daughter to translate for her. The daughter translates the screening questions for depression and the responses to the two questions are positive.

▶ *What may be the causes of her worsening diabetes control and how should you respond to the positive responses to the screening questions for depression?*

Cultural and ethnic considerations

There is a fourfold increased risk of Type 2 diabetes amongst people from South Asia (Indians, Sri Lankans, Pakistanis and Bangladeshis) living in the UK as compared with Europeans.[1] Type 2 diabetes also seems to develop in South Asians about 10 years earlier than in Europeans, and renal and cardiac complications are encountered more commonly.

Although genetic factors are important, the increased risk of Type 2 diabetes is strongly associated with increasing central obesity and insulin resistance.

The particular educational needs of the South Asian community need to be addressed, with the creation of programmes on healthy lifestyle, improved diet and increased physical activity. These programmes are designed to reduce obesity and hence lessen the risks of developing Type 2 diabetes. They need to be culturally sensitive and be available in appropriate languages; the use of Asian link workers to promote such programmes is being tested in some areas of the UK. Similar educational interventions need to be provided for South Asian people who develop Type 2 diabetes. Translators may be needed to assist in consultations with people who cannot speak English.

The United Kingdom Asian Diabetes Study (UKADS), a community-based intervention in South Asian people with Type 2 diabetes, is testing the hypothesis that a 'structured culturally sensitive care package tailored to the needs of the South Asian community will improve cardiovascular risk factors and ultimately morbidity and mortality in a cost-effective manner'. The care package being evaluated was additional practice nurse time, supported by link workers and input from a diabetes specialist nurse. In a pilot study conducted in six inner-city practices the intervention produced significant improvements in blood pressure and total cholesterol measurements after one year, but no change in Hb_{A1c} levels, compared with a control group.[2]

Care during Ramadan

The decision on whether to fast during Ramadan is a decision to be made by the patient with diabetes. The length of the fast (from sunrise to sunset) will vary according to the time of the year in which Ramadan falls. The maximum length occurs if Ramadan falls in the summer months, when it may last for 18 hours. Most people with well-controlled diabetes should be able to fast safely.[3] Fasting may be judged to be unsafe in some individuals with brittle diabetes, or those with cardiac and renal complications. If fasting is deemed to be medically detrimental a person can be exempted from fasting. Some people may want reassurance from their religious authorities when deciding not to fast.

It is advisable to eat foods high in dietary fibre such as whole grains, fruits and vegetables at the pre-dawn and sunset meals to promote good glycaemic control.

People on diet control and those taking metformin, glitazone or a dipeptidyl peptidase-4 (DPP-4) inhibitor, or combinations of these, are at very low risk of hypoglycaemia and so should have no problems.

If the patient is taking a long-acting sulphonylurea drug it is better to change to a shorter-acting one to avoid the risk of hypoglycaemia during the day.

People on once-daily insulin could consider switching to a twice-daily pre-mix regime during Ramadan. Those on twice-daily could consider taking half the evening dose before dawn and the normal morning dose at sunset. Those on basal bolus therapy could reduce the long-acting component and miss out on the middle-of-the-day short-acting component.

More self-monitoring of blood glucose (SMBG) testing should be carried out to guide alterations in insulin and sulphonylurea therapy. More detailed advice may need to be obtained in those on insulin, especially people on basal bolus regimes.

It is important to emphasise the need to carry glucose tablets during the day and that it is legitimate to break the fast in emergency situations, e.g. a hypoglycaemia episode.

Social and workplace issues

Diabetes UK

Diabetes UK is a charity for people with diabetes, for those who care for them and for healthcare professionals involved in delivering diabetes care. It provides information about all aspects of diabetes, has a care line that can be phoned for information and advice, and raises money for research in diabetes. The charity has a head office in London, offices in most of the regions, and supports local groups in many areas of the UK.[4] Diabetes UK is the main source of advice and help for all social and workplace issues related to diabetes.

Driving

Hypoglycaemia is a risk for people with diabetes treated with insulin or agents that stimulate the release of insulin. A hypoglycaemia episode that occurs when driving may cause a road traffic accident. There is therefore a requirement for people with diabetes to inform the Driver and Vehicle Licensing Agency (DVLA) of their condition. Full details can be found in the DVLA publication on the medical aspects of fitness to drive.[5] A brief summary of the main recommendations is as follows.

INSULIN-TREATED DIABETES

The patient:

▷ must inform the DVLA and insurance company
▷ can hold a normal driving licence (group 1) but will not be eligible for a group 2 (large goods vehicles and passenger-carrying vehicles).

ORAL AGENT-TREATED DIABETES

The patient:

▷ must inform the DVLA and insurance company
▷ can hold a group 1 licence
▷ may hold a group 2 licence subject to satisfactory medical review.

DIET AND EXERCISE ALONE

▷ There are no restrictions; the patient does not need to inform the DVLA.

Patients on insulin therapy are advised to check blood glucose levels before starting to drive and ensure that they take snacks to eat. They are advised to pull over and stop driving if any symptoms suggestive of impending hypoglycaemia occur. Loss of hypoglycaemic awareness and frequent hypoglycaemic episodes should lead to cessation of driving until the problem is resolved.

Employment issues

People with diabetes can and should be encouraged to undertake a wide variety of employment. There are however restrictions in some occupations where hypoglycaemia would pose a risk to the person with diabetes, their working colleagues or members of the general public.

Patients treated with insulin

These are not usually accepted for employment in the armed services, the police, the merchant navy, the fire brigade, the prison service, deep-sea diving, working on oil rigs, heavy commercial goods driving, bus driving, underground mining, or as pilots or in air traffic control.

If patients develop diabetes and require insulin treatment whilst employed in one of the above occupations they will normally have to stop their work. However, as indicated below, Diabetes UK fights for individual assessment of risk, rather than blanket bans.

Patients on diet or diet and tablets

Those treated with diet alone, or on diet and oral medications, can undertake most occupations as the risk of hypoglycaemia is small.

Some of the employment restrictions encountered in the UK may have been established by individual companies or industries rather than by legislation. Diabetes UK campaigns for individual assessment of risk in employment, taking into account the type and method of diabetes treatment, rather than blanket bans.

Travel

Patients with diabetes should experience few problems with long-distance travel providing they have planned properly. It is important to declare diabetes when obtaining quotations for travel insurance to ensure appropriate cover.

Insulin and accessories should be carried in hand luggage. Insulin will freeze and be rendered ineffective if kept in luggage stored in the cargo hold of an aircraft. In these times of high security a written statement from a healthcare professional confirming diabetes and the need to carry insulin, accessories and needles is helpful. Also, the extended day that occurs during a long westward aeroplane flight may require an additional dose of short-acting insulin with a meal on board the aircraft.

Insulin absorption may be increased in hot climates. This may result in an increased risk of hypoglycaemia, which patients with insulin-treated diabetes need to be aware of. There is also a risk of damage to insensitive feet from walking on hot sand, and people with such at-risk feet should be warned to wear protective footwear in hot climates.

Alcohol

Alcohol can be taken in moderation by patients who have diabetes. The maximum recommendations are three units a day for men and two units a day for women. Alcohol lowers blood glucose levels, so it is important for people with diabetes not to drink on an empty stomach. *Alcohol abuse is dangerous in people with diabetes because hypoglycaemia can pass undetected in inebriated people.*

Depression

The overall prevalence of depression in Type 2 diabetes is similar to that observed in other chronic diseases, and is greater than matched populations without diabetes. Being diagnosed with diabetes imposes a lifelong psychological burden on the patient and his or her family. Poor psychological functioning causes suffering, can seriously interfere with daily diabetes self-management, and is associated with poor medical outcomes and high healthcare costs.[6,7]

It is important therefore to detect depression so that it can be treated.

Depression and the Quality and Outcomes Framework

A new clinical indicator DEP1 was introduced in 2006/7. It states:

The percentage of patients on the diabetes register and/or the CHD [chronic heart disease] register for whom case finding for depression has been undertaken on one occasion during the previous 15 months using two standard screening questions.

Minimum threshold = 40%: maximum threshold to earn full available 8 points = 90%.

Two screening questions that need to be asked of everyone with diabetes are:

1 ▷ During the last month, have you often been bothered by feeling down, depressed or hopeless?
2 ▷ During the last month, have you often been bothered by having little interest or pleasure in doing things?

A yes answer to either question is considered a positive response.

The concept of screening high-risk groups that include patients with diabetes and patients with CHD for depression is from the NICE Clinical Guideline for the management of depression.[8]

There is evidence that treating depression in patients with diabetes with antidepressant medications can improve depression but does not improve Hb_{A1c}. There is an evidence base for fluoxetine.[9] A recent systematic review and meta-analysis has shown that, overall, psychological interventions are effective in improving glycaemic control in Type 2 diabetes.[10]

If depression is detected using the screening questions a consultation needs to take place between the healthcare professional and the patient with diabetes to discuss the background, causation, associated factors, severity and need for treatment. Treatment options may include antidepressant medications and counselling and talking therapies.

Scenario revisited

You discover that Jaswinder has been fasting for Ramadan, which finished 4 weeks ago. She says that she felt tired and weak around midday when she was fasting, so she stopped all her tablets and has not restarted them.

Her daughter says that her mum is feeling depressed because her husband has been away in Pakistan on family business for the past 2 months.

You explain the importance of restarting the metformin and gliclazide medications, and arrange for the Asian link worker, who speaks her first language, to visit her at home to discuss her medications, her positive answers to the depression screening questions and the need to manage her medications in a different way during the next period of Ramadan.

Summary

In relation to the six domains of core or essential competences of being a GP:

1 Primary care management

▷ Recognition of the need to consider modification of treatment in Ramadan if hypoglycaemia is a possible complication of fasting.
▷ Recognition and management of depression in the context of a chronic disease like diabetes.

2 Person-centred care

▷ To be aware of the impact psycho-social issues may have on the individual living with diabetes.

3 Specific problem-solving skills

▷ Understanding of the issues of diabetes and driving to enable the healthcare professional and patient with diabetes to consent to appropriate therapeutic choices for treating glycaemia.

4 A comprehensive approach

▷ Consideration of the physical, psychological and social issues relating to diabetes.
▷ The need to be aware of cultural issues and being sensitive to these, and employing interpreters where appropriate to facilitate effective communication and a shared understanding.

5 Community orientation

▷ To be aware of the help that Diabetes UK can give to patients with diabetes in issues relating to employment and insurance.

6 A holistic approach

▷ To understand the impact of diabetes on all aspects of daily living including travel, employment and insurance.
▷ To understand how depression may accompany diabetes as a chronic disease, and the impact it can have.

Useful websites

Diabetes UK • **www.diabetes.org.uk**.
DVLA • **www.dvla.gov.uk**.

References

1 • Choudhury T A, Grace C, Kopelman P. Preventing diabetes in South Asians (editorial) *British Medical Journal* 2003; **327**: 1059–60.

2 • O'Hare J P, Raymond N T, Mughal S, *et al.* Evaluation of delivery of enhanced diabetes care to patients of South Asian ethnicity: the United Kingdom Asian Diabetes Study (UKADS) *Diabetic Medicine* 2004; **21**: 1357–65.

3 • Sheikh A, Wallia S. Ramadan fasting and diabetes *British Medical Journal* 2007; **335**: 613–14.

4 • www.diabetes.org.uk [accessed July 2009].

5 • Drivers Medical Group, DVLA. *For Medical Practitioners: at a glance guide to the current medical standards of fitness to drive* DVLA: Swansea, www.dvla.gov.uk/medical/ataglance. aspx [accessed July 2009].

6 • Lin E H, Katon W, Von Korff M, *et al.* Relationship of depression and diabetes self-care, medication adherence, and preventive care *Diabetes Care* 2004; **27**: 2154–60.

7 • Egede L E, Zheng P, Simpson K. Comorbid depression is associated with increased health care use and expenditure in individuals with diabetes *Diabetes Care* 2002; **25**: 464–70.

8 • National Institute for Health and Clinical Excellence. *Clinical Guideline 23, Depression: management of depression in primary and secondary care* London: NICE, 2004, www.nice.org. uk/CG023 [accessed July 2009].

9 • Lustman P J, Freedland K E, Griffith L S, *et al.* Fluoxetine for depression in diabetes: a randomized double blind placebo controlled trial *Diabetes Care* 2000; **23**: 618–23.

10 • Ismail K, Winkley K, Rabe-Hesketh S. Systematic review and meta-analysis of randomized controlled trials of psychological interventions to improve glycaemic control in patients with type 2 diabetes *Lancet* 2004; **363**: 1589–97.

Structures of care for diabetes patients

8

Scenario

Alison is a 27-year-old woman who has had Type 1 diabetes for 12 years. She is on a basal bolus insulin regime and went on a dose adjustment for normal eating (DAFNE) course 3 years ago. She has two children, aged 2 and 4, and looks after them full time. She has no diabetes complications. She has not been to the hospital clinic since her youngest child was born as she says she is too busy with her two small children. She attends the surgery for a 'pill' check and asks if she can have an update of her insulin prescription. None of the annual review fields has been filled in on the practice diabetes template for the Quality and Outcomes Framework (QoF).

▶ *How would you manage her request?*

Shift of diabetes from secondary care to primary care

Until around 20 to 30 years ago diabetes was seen as a condition to be managed wholly by a hospital-based specialist. Over the past 20 to 30 years increasing numbers of people have been diagnosed with diabetes, which has meant that the hospital specialist model has come under considerable strain. In the UK this was highlighted in a report from the Audit Commission entitled *Testing Times*, which reviewed secondary care diabetes services and concluded that many services were greatly stretched. One way forward proposed in the report was for primary care to provide more of the routine care so that hospitals could concentrate on specialist care and professional support and training, while allowing patients to receive continuity of care closer to home.[1]

In the UK there has been a gradual shift in thinking over the past 10 to 20 years and now diabetes is seen as a condition that should be largely managed in primary care. The QoF of the new GP contract introduced in 2004 has provided encouragement and incentive for primary care to take on this work.

New GP contract Quality and Outcomes Framework

The diabetes clinical area of the new contract, for the first 2 years 2004/5 and 2005/6, had a maximum of 99 points (approximately 10 per cent of the total points available) spread across 18 clinical indicators). The only other clinical area with more points (121) was that of coronary heart disease (CHD) including left ventricular dysfunction (LVD). This indicated the importance of diabetes.

The results for the first 2 years showed an increase in points scored for both the process of care indicators and the quality of care indicators (see Table 8.1).

Table 8.1 ○ *Achievement of diabetes clinical indicators in the QoF 2004/5 and 2005/6*

Quality indicator		2005/6			2004/5	Difference
		Denominator	Numerator	%	%	
DM2	The percentage of patients with diabetes whose notes record BMI in the previous 15 months	1,835,480	1,726,599	94.1	90.6	3.5
DM3	The percentage of patients with diabetes in whom there is a record of smoking status in the previous 15 months except those who have never smoked where smoking status should be recorded once	1,870,940	1,821,376	97.4	95.9	1.5
DM4	The percentage of patients with diabetes who smoke and whose notes contain a record that smoking cessation advice has been offered in the last 15 months	277,317	265,623	95.8	93.2	2.6
DM5	The percentage of diabetic patients who have a record of Hb_{A1c} or equivalent in the previous 15 months	1,841,571	1,776,415	96.5	94.4	2.1

Quality indicator	2005/6			2004/5	Difference
	Denominator	Numerator	%	%	
DM6 The percentage of patients with diabetes in whom the last Hb$_{A1c}$ is 7.4 or less (or equivalent test/ reference range depending on local laboratory) in last 15 months	1,674,231	1,034,293	61.8	58.8	3.0
DM7 The percentage of patients with diabetes in whom the last Hb$_{A1c}$ is 10 or less (or equivalent test/ reference range depending on local laboratory) in last 15 months	1,786,114	1,633,981	91.5	89.4	2.1
DM8 The percentage of patients with diabetes who have a record of retinal screening in the previous 15 months	1,781,716	1,580,830	88.7	83.4	5.3
DM9 The percentage of patients with diabetes with a record of presence or absence of peripheral pulses in the previous 15 months	1,785,322	1,574,374	88.2	78.9	9.3
DM10 The percentage of patients with diabetes with a record of neuropathy testing in the previous 15 months	1,782,667	1,558,411	87.4	77.6	9.8
DM11 The percentage of patients with diabetes who have a record of the blood pressure in the past 15 months	1,874,539	1,840,954	98.2	97.0	1.2
DM12 The percentage of patients with diabetes in whom the last blood pressure is 145/85 or less	1,753,856	1,313,740	74.9	70.3	4.6

Quality indicator	2005/6			2004/5	Difference
	Denominator	Numerator	%	%	
DM13 The percentage of patients with diabetes who have a record of microalbuminuria testing in the previous 15 months (exception reporting for patients with proteinuria)	1,684,327	1,396,760	82.9	70.9	12.0
DM14 The percentage of patients with diabetes who have a record of serum creatinine testing in the previous 15 months	1,857,309	1,777,422	95.7	93.0	2.7
DM15 The percentage of patients with diabetes with proteinuria or microalbuminuria who are treated with ACE inhibitors (or A2 antagonists)	161,211	138,292	85.8	82.1	3.7
DM16 The percentage of patients with diabetes who have a record of total cholesterol in the previous 15 months	1,849,405	1,764,280	95.4	92.7	2.7
DM17 The percentage of patients with diabetes whose last measured total cholesterol within previous 15 months is 5 or less	1,703,389	1,345,409	79.0	71.8	7.2
DM18 The percentage of patients with diabetes who have had influenza immunisation in the preceding 1 September to 31 March	1,651,515	1,477,561	89.5	85.2	4.3
Diabetes prevalence (registered)	53,211,253	1,890,663	3.6	3.4	0.2

Source: copyright © the Health and Social Care Information Centre.

Table 8.2 ○ *Changes in diabetes indicators for 2006/7*

Diabetes mellitus (diabetes)

Indicator		Points	Threshold	Points	Threshold
Records					
DM1	The practice can produce a register of all patients with diabetes mellitus	6			Moved to DM19
DM19	The practice can produce a register of all patients aged 17 years and over with diabetes mellitus, which specifies whether the patient has Type 1 or Type 2 diabetes	Moved from DM1		6	
Ongoing management					
DM2	The percentage of patients with diabetes whose notes record BMI in the previous 15 months	3	25–90%	3	40–90%
DM3	The percentage of patients with diabetes in whom there is a record of smoking status in the previous 15 months except those who have never smoked where smoking status should be recorded once	3	25–90%		Moved to SMOKING
DM4	The percentage of patients with diabetes who smoke and whose notes contain a record that smoking cessation advice has been offered in the last 15 months	5	25–90%		
DM5	The percentage of diabetic patients who have a record of Hb_{A1c} or equivalent in the previous 15 months	6	25–90%		40–90%

87

Indicator		Points	Threshold	Points	Threshold
DM6	The percentage of patients with diabetes in whom the last Hb_{A1c} is 7.4 or less (or equivalent test/ reference range depending on local laboratory) in last 15 months	16	25–50%	Moved to DM20	
DM20	The percentage of patients with diabetes in whom the last Hb_{A1c} is 7.5 or less (or equivalent test/ reference range depending on local laboratory) in the previous 15 months	Moved from DM6		17	40–50%
DM7	The percentage of patients with diabetes in whom the last Hb_{A1c} is 10 or less (or equivalent test/ reference range depending on local laboratory) in last 15 months	11	25–85%	11	40–90%
DM8	The percentage of patients with diabetes who have a record of retinal screening in the previous 15 months	5	25–90%	Moved to DM21	
DM21	The percentage of patients with diabetes who have a record of retinal screening in the previous 15 months	Moved from DM8		5	40–90%
DM9	The percentage of patients with diabetes with a record of presence or absence of peripheral pulses in the previous 15 months	3	25–90%	3	40–90%
DM10	The percentage of patients with diabetes with a record of neuropathy testing in the previous 15 months	3	25–90%	3	40–90%

Indicator		Points	Threshold	Points	Threshold
DM11	The percentage of patients with diabetes who have a record of the blood pressure in the past 15 months	3	25–90%	3	40–90%
DM12	The percentage of patients with diabetes in whom the last blood pressure is 145/85 or less	3	25–90%	3	40–90%
DM13	The percentage of patients with diabetes who have a record of microalbuminuria testing in the previous 15 months (exception reporting for patients with proteinuria)	3	25–90%	3	40–90%
DM14	The percentage of patients with diabetes who have a record of serum creatinine testing in the previous 15 months	3	25–90%	Moved to DM22	
DM22	The percentage of patients with diabetes who have a record of estimated glomerular filtration rate (eGFR) or serum creatinine testing in the previous 15 months	Moved from DM14		3	40–90%
DM15	The percentage of patients with diabetes with proteinuria or microalbuminuria who are treated with ACE inhibitors (or A2 antagonists)	3	25–70%	3	40–80%
DM16	The percentage of patients with diabetes who have a record of total cholesterol in the previous 15 months	3	25–90%	3	40–90%
DM17	The percentage of patients with diabetes whose last measured total cholesterol within previous 15 months is 5 or less	6	25–60%	6	40–70%

Indicator		Points	Threshold	Points	Threshold
DM18	The percentage of patients with diabetes who have had influenza immunisation in the preceding 1 September to 31 March	3	25–85%	3	40–85%

Depression

Indicator		Points	Threshold	Points	Threshold
Diagnosis and initial management					
DEP1	The percentage of patients on the diabetes register and/ or the CHD register for whom case finding for depression has been undertaken on one occasion during the previous 15 months using two standard screening questions			8	40–90%

Source: copyright© the Health and Social Care Information Centre.

For the years 2006/7 and 2007/8 there were a maximum of 93 points for the clinical indicators (see Table 8.3).

Table 8.3 ○ *Achievement of the diabetes clinical indicators in 2006/7*

Indicator	Points available	Total points achieved	Total points achieved/available %	Underlying achievement
DM19	6	49,740.0	100.0%	—
DM2	3	24,638.9	99.0%	94.9%
DM5	3	24,775.5	99.6%	97.1%
DM20	17	138,595.4	98.3%	66.8%
DM7	11	89,308.2	97.9%	92.3%
DM21	5	38,783.1	93.5%	90.2%
DM9	3	23,640.6	95.0%	91.1%
DM10	3	23,541.8	94.6%	90.8%
DM11	3	24,851.9	99.9%	98.5%
DM12	18	148,671.7	99.6%	79.3%
DM13	3	22,275.4	89.5%	86.5%
DM22	3	24,762.6	99.5%	96.8%
DM15	3	23,866.4	95.9%	89.1%
DM16	3	24,749.5	99.5%	96.1%
DM17	6	49,387.2	99.2%	83.2%
DM18	3	24,461.9	98.3%	90.4%
Diabetes total	93	756,050.1	98.0%	

Source: copyright© the Health and Social Care Information Centre.

There has been an improvement in the diabetes process and quality of care indicators in each of the years of the 2004 GP contract.

GPs with a Special Interest in diabetes

In the UK the government is encouraging the development of the concept of the GP with a Special Interest (GPwSI) to help facilitate care of chronic disease in the community. The idea is that a full-time GP may take up to 1 day a week to work as a GPwSI in a specific clinical field. Framework documents for the work of GPwSIs have been published.[2] GPwSIs in diabetes could fulfil a purely management function, for example overseeing a diabetes network, or could fulfil a clinical function, for example running diabetes clinics in the community for people with diabetes whose problems have not been successfully managed in general practice.

This concept of setting up community or intermediate clinics staffed by GPwSIs, community diabetologists (doctors trained as specialists in diabetes but who are now working in the community), community-based diabetes specialist nurses, podiatrists, dieticians and others as necessary, has been pioneered in several areas in the UK. The idea is that most routine diabetes care is given at practice level, but where the practice does not have the skills to deal with specific, more complex, problems the patient can be seen in an intermediate clinic nearer to his or her home, rather than having to travel to a hospital out-patient clinic. Examples of such problems include the need to initiate insulin in someone with Type 2 diabetes who is not adequately controlled on oral therapy, or the patient whose hyperlipidaemia is not controlled on statin therapy alone.

Primary care diabetes team

This should consist of a motivated general practitioner (primary care physician) and practice nurse(s) with special training in diabetes care. They should have access to a team of healthcare professionals including dietician, podiatrist and a diabetes nurse or district (community) nurse with well-defined responsibilities for each team member. They should work closely with local community pharmacists.

The practice should have a dedicated record-keeping system and a diabetes disease register, with quality assessment and a recall system to enhance clinic attendance. There should also be a structured protocol to include criteria for referral to a hospital specialist.

Running a diabetes clinic in the practice

Staff and dedicated diabetes time

Many practices in the UK run diabetes clinics in which practice nurses with special training and expertise in diabetes care recall and review patients with diabetes. Such clinics are supervised by the GP partner in the practice with an interest in diabetes care.

Healthcare assistants (HCAs) are now being employed by a number of practices. They can help in diabetes clinics by collecting and recording some of the clinical information, e.g. weight, blood pressure and foot screening, leaving the practice diabetes nurse more time to spend on education and support. In practices with small numbers of people with diabetes, dedicated diabetes clinics may be impractical and dedicated diabetes time may be best provided in special slots in ordinary surgery times. It is vital that staff providing diabetes care are appropriately skilled. There is a number of excellent diabetes education and training programmes that are available in the UK, which enable healthcare professionals to gain certification of training through certificates, diplomas and masters degrees in diabetes. One example is the Certificate in Diabetes Care (CIDC) from the University of Warwick, which is a five-and-a-half-day taught programme delivered over 6 months. Over 6000 GPs and practice nurses have successfully completed the programme.[3]

A number of universities have masters programmes in diabetes for those who wish to study diabetes at this level.

The Primary Care Diabetes Society (PCDS) has been set up as a national group to offer support and encouragement to community diabetes teams. It has an annual conference and other educational events.[4] The journal *Diabetes and Primary Care* contains specific pages dedicated to the Society.

Diabetes register

One of the basic building blocks for running such a clinic is a diabetes register. In the vast majority of practices in the UK this is an electronic register. The register prevalence of diabetes from the 2006/7 QoF database is 3.7 per cent. Figures below 3.7 per cent in practices with 'average' ethnicity and an 'average' age distribution imply under-recording or under-diagnosis. In practices with many people from ethnic minority backgrounds the practice prevalence may rise to 8–12 per cent. Inaccuracies may occur in the practice diabetes register and the following are possible causes of inaccuracy:

1 ▷ People diagnosed as having diabetes many years ago, simply through having glycosuria, being included on the register. When their notes are inspected it is found that no diagnostic blood tests were ever performed
2 ▷ People with gestational diabetes being put on the diabetes register
3 ▷ People with diabetes insipidus being put on the register
4 ▷ People with impaired fasting glucose (IFG) or impaired glucose tolerance (IGT) being wrongly labelled as having diabetes and being put on the register.

PEOPLE WITH POSSIBLE DIABETES LYING UNDETECTED IN THE PRACTICE CLINICAL DATABASE

Holt *et al.*[5] inform us of the worrying statistic that around 1 per cent of the UK population has diabetes that is undiagnosed or unrecorded on practice disease registers. When the computer records of 3.6 million patients were searched from 480 GP practices it was found that the last blood glucose level in approximately 0.1 per cent was indicative of undiagnosed diabetes, and that for 0.9 per cent the last blood glucose level was at best borderline, leaving many at risk of diabetes or having undiagnosed diabetes. Also only one third of people aged over 40 years without diabetes have had their blood glucose measured in the past 2 years. Therefore it is important that people with borderline glucose readings enter a system for recall and dietary intervention, and perhaps a great proportion of the over-40s are screened.

CLINIC TEMPLATE

Practice clinical computer systems contain a diabetes clinic template that automatically uses the appropriate Read codes for recording care. These are updated each year to ensure that they record care information by designated Read codes in a form that will fit the quality indicators from the new contract. A diabetes dataset has been developed and is being modified to allow accurate recording of the various items of clinical care that need to be recorded to document care for the contract quality payments. In most GP practices diabetes care blood tests are requested 2 weeks before clinic attendance, so that this information is available on the clinic day. Many systems receive test results from the local laboratory by electronic download. These test results are then posted into the diabetes clinical template.

FREQUENCY OF REVIEW

This clearly depends on the needs of the particular individual. When someone is newly diagnosed the patient's clinical condition may mean that he or she needs reviewing very frequently until glycaemic control is optimised. Once a patient is stabilised and targets for glycaemia and blood pressure have been optimised routine review every 6 months is usual.

Many GPs who have undertaken post-qualification diabetes training are able with their diabetes practice team to look after most of the patients with diabetes in the practice. There are however a number of situations in which referral to specialist secondary care is important.

Suggested criteria for referral to specialist secondary care

These criteria are:

▷ children or teenagers newly diagnosed with diabetes
▷ women with diabetes contemplating pregnancy
▷ women with diabetes who are pregnant
▷ people with severe vascular complications
▷ people who require treatment for diabetic eye disease, foot ulceration
  or nephropathy
▷ people with unstable cardiovascular disease
▷ people with poor metabolic control where it is proving very difficult
  to control Hb_{A1c}, lipids or blood pressure to agreed targets.

Practice-Based Commissioning

Practice-Based Commissioning (PBC) initiatives are being developed to assist in further improving diabetes care in the community. A diabetes commissioning toolkit has been developed to assist commissioning consortia.[6] The National Institute for Health and Clinical Excellence (NICE) has developed a commissioning document for diabetes foot care based on the NICE guidelines from 2004 to enable the recommended levels of foot care provision to be commissioned.[7,8]

In a number of areas diabetes services are being redesigned through PBC initiatives. Some areas have developed 'intermediate clinics' in the community, often staffed by community diabetes specialist nurses and GPwSIs (or occasionally community diabetologists). These clinics receive referrals from practices that might otherwise have had to send patients to secondary care out-patient clinics.

Some areas have developed locally enhanced services (LES) for diabetes. These can provide the financial support to enable practices to initiate insulin in patients with Type 2 diabetes, rather than having to refer to secondary care.

Scenario revisited

You need to gently negotiate with Alison a minimum level of supervision of her diabetes that will enable her to be confident that she is well-controlled and has no developing complications. She agrees to attend the practice once a year for an annual review consultation, having agreed to have a blood test a couple of weeks before, as long as the consultation can be at a time when she can get someone to look after her children.

You agree to this and write to the local diabetologist explaining that this is happening.

You gently raise the subject of family planning, noting that she is happy taking the oral contraceptive, and suggest that if in the future she is thinking of having another child she comes to discuss pre-conception issues with you.

Summary

In relation to the six domains of core or essential competences of being a GP:

1 Primary care management

▷ Understanding the QoF clinical indicators and developing structured processes of care in the practice with a diabetes disease register and appropriate training of staff.

2 Person-centred care

▷ Being sensitive to the individual needs of people with diabetes and having flexibility in the practice diabetes provision to allow for individual needs. This may vary according to the size of practice. Smaller practices may have individual sessions rather than 'clinics'.

3 Specific problem-solving skills

▷ To be able to discuss and negotiate a minimum of an annual review for someone with diabetes.

4 A comprehensive approach

▷ To be able to provide diabetes care in the context of any other healthcare needs of the individual, ensuring that medication updates and review of other co-morbidities take place together.

5 Community orientation

▷ To encourage the individual to get support and help from others with diabetes by attending the local Diabetes UK support group.

6 A holistic approach

▷ To understand the impact that attending for review of diabetes has on the individual, his or her family and work.

Useful websites

Primary Care Diabetes Society • **www.pcdsociety.org**.

References

1 • Audit Commission. *Testing Times: a review of diabetes services in England and Wales* London: Audit Commission, 2000.

2 • Department of Health. *Implementing Care Closer to Home: convenient quality care for patients. Part 3: the accreditation of GPs and pharmacists with special interests* London: DoH, 2007, www.dh.gov.uk/en/Healthcare/Primarycare/Practitionerswithspecialinterests/DH_074419 [accessed July 2009].

3 • www2.warwick.ac.uk/fac/med/study/cpd/subject_index/diabetes/ for continuing professional development courses in diabetes from the University of Warwick [accessed July 2009].

4 • www.pcdsociety.org [accessed July 2009].

5 • Holt T A, Stables D, Hippisley-Cox J, *et al*. Identifying undiagnosed diabetes: cross-sectional survey of 3.6 million patients' electronic records *British Journal of General Practice* 2008; **58(548)**: 192–6.

6 • Department of Health. *Diabetes Commissioning Toolkit* London: DoH, 2006, www.dh.gov.uk/en/Publicationsandstatistics/Publications/PublicationsPolicyAndGuidance/DH_4140284 [accessed July 2009].

7 • National Institute for Clinical Excellence. *Clinical Guideline 10, Prevention and Management of Foot Problems in Type 2 Diabetes* London: NICE, 2004, www.nice.org.uk/nicemedia/pdf/CG010NICEguideline.pdf [accessed July 2009].

8 • National Institute for Health and Clinical Excellence. *Commissioning Guide for Diabetes Footcare* London: NICE, 2006, www.nice.org.uk/usingguidance/commissioningguides/footcare/foot_care_service_for_people_with_diabetes.jsp [accessed July 2009].

Diabetes and pregnancy

Introduction – the increased risks

Women with Type 1 and Type 2 diabetes have an increased risk of adverse pregnancy outcomes including:

▷ miscarriage
▷ foetal congenital anomaly
▷ perinatal death.[1]

There is a significant relationship between adverse outcomes of pregnancy and poor glycaemic control in early pregnancy in women with diabetes. In one UK study of women with Type 1 diabetes[2] there was a fourfold increase in adverse outcomes, a fourfold increase in spontaneous abortion and a ninefold increase in major malformation in women with an Hb_{A1c} above 7.5 per cent at booking.

Reducing the risks

There is evidence that the infants of women with diabetes who attend multidisciplinary pre-pregnancy counselling show significantly fewer major congenital malformations compared with infants of non-attending mothers. The attending mothers also have fewer pregnancy complications.[3]

There is good evidence that optimal blood glucose control before and during pregnancy reduces congenital malformations, stillbirth, neonatal hypoglycaemia and respiratory distress syndrome. Blood glucose levels around conception should be as normal as possible, with a target Hb_{A1c} of below 6.1 per cent. This is likely to require intensive blood glucose monitoring and intensive insulin therapy in many people.[4]

Pregnancy and women with diabetes

Around 650,000 women give birth in England and Wales each year, and 2–5 per cent of pregnancies involve women with diabetes.[4]

Pregnancy care in women with diabetes used to relate almost exclusively to women with Type 1 diabetes, as Type 2 diabetes was only seen in older people – outside of the reproductive years.

Type 2 diabetes is now being diagnosed in teenagers in the UK, most of whom are significantly obese. It is likely therefore that pregnancy in women with Type 2 diabetes who may be treated with diet alone, or diet and metformin, or diet, metformin and other oral agents, will become more common, and this is now being seen in the UK.

So now pre-existing Type 1 diabetes and pre-existing Type 2 diabetes are felt to account for 0.27 per cent and 0.10 per cent of births, respectively, in the UK.[4]

NICE guideline on pregnancy and diabetes

The National Institute for Health and Clinical Excellence (NICE) published its first guideline on diabetes in pregnancy in 2008.[4] This reviews the management of diabetes from pre-conception to the postnatal period, and makes a large number of recommendations. Most of the care for pregnant women with diabetes will be provided in secondary care, and therefore many of the recommendations have specific relevance there. However, it contains several important recommendations that need to be implemented in primary care.

The role of primary care

Most women with Type 1 diabetes have been looked after in secondary care. It has been the responsibility of secondary care professionals to ensure that women are referred to pre-conception clinics when planning pregnancy. It may have been felt that primary care had a slight responsibility to ensure that women with diabetes who planned to become pregnant were referred to such pre-conception clinics, but it was not felt it had the responsibility to deliver pre-conception advice. However, it is important to state that women with diabetes cannot be divided into a group planning to become pregnant and a group not planning to become pregnant. In one study of women with Type 1 diabetes 40 per cent had not planned the pregnancy.[1] This may also be true for those with Type 2 diabetes.

Women are being diagnosed with Type 2 diabetes in childbearing age and may be being looked after exclusively in primary care. Pre-conception advice for this group will therefore have to be provided in primary care.

Recommendations from the NICE guideline on pre-conception care for women with diabetes

▷ Women with diabetes should be informed about the benefits of pre-conception glycaemic control at each contact with healthcare professionals, including their diabetes care team, from adolescence.

▷ The intentions of women with diabetes regarding pregnancy and contraceptive use should be documented at each contact with their diabetes care team.

▷ The importance of avoiding unplanned pregnancy should be an essential component of diabetes education from adolescence for women with diabetes.

▷ Stop angiotensin-converting enzyme (ACE) inhibitors and angiotensin II (AT2) receptor antagonists and statins if these are being prescribed for women with diabetes, as these medications can cause congenital malformations.

101

The role of primary care

Primary care is in contact with women with pre-existing diabetes through the provision of contraception, the prescription of diabetes repeat medications, and the treatment of acute illness. All these contacts need to be used to reinforce the messages in the above recommendations. GPs and practice nurses providing contraceptive advice, repeat medication reviews, and diabetes clinics need to be aware of these recommendations and to take every opportunity to reinforce the messages of pregnancy planning and the importance of good glycaemic control at conception and in pregnancy.

All women with diabetes need to be referred to specialist care as soon as possible after they become pregnant for intensive blood glucose control and monitoring throughout pregnancy and delivery.

This specialist care needs to be provided through good co-operation between a diabetologist with an interest in pregnancy and an obstetrician with a special interest in diabetes, who run joint clinics to care for women with diabetes throughout their pregnancies. Such team-working facilitates appropriate diabetes and obstetric considerations to be taken into account throughout the pregnancy, together with appropriate liaison with the primary healthcare team.

Gestational diabetes

Gestational diabetes (GDM) is carbohydrate intolerance with onset or first recognition during pregnancy. It includes women with abnormal glucose tolerance that reverts to normal after pregnancy, and those with Type 1 and Type 2 diabetes newly diagnosed in pregnancy.

There is an up to 50 per cent risk of future diabetes in women who develop GDM, and babies of mothers with GDM have an increased risk of perinatal morbidity.

The NICE guideline development group estimates that 87.5 per cent of pregnancies complicated with diabetes are due to GDM and 7.5 per cent due to Type 1 diabetes. The remaining 5 per cent are due to Type 2 diabetes.[4]

A recent high-quality randomised controlled trial has shown that diagnosis and intervention for gestational diabetes improves maternal and foetal outcomes.[5]

The NICE guideline group therefore recommends that screening for gestational diabetes using risk factors is carried out at the booking appointment. A standard oral glucose tolerance test (OGTT) at 24–28 weeks should be the screening test that is used. Women with previous GDM should receive an OGTT at 16–18 weeks followed by one at 28 weeks if the first test is normal.

The group states also that:

▷ hypoglycaemic therapy should be considered for women with gestational diabetes if diet and exercise fail to maintain blood glucose targets during a period of 1–2 weeks
▷ hypoglycaemic therapy (which may include insulin and/or metformin and glibenclamide) should be tailored to the glycaemic profile of, and acceptability to, the individual pregnant women.

Follow-up of women with gestational diabetes mellitus

Women who have had GDM in a pregnancy have a 10-year risk of 50 per cent of developing Type 2 diabetes, and also are likely to develop GDM in any subsequent pregnancy. The NICE guideline[4] states that women who have had GDM should receive advice on:

▷ weight control, diet and exercise
▷ the symptoms of hyperglycaemia
▷ the risks of GDM in subsequent pregnancies and screening for diabetes when planning pregnancy.

Women with GDM should be offered:

▷ a blood glucose test before transfer into community care
▷ a fasting glucose test at the 6-week postnatal appointment, then
   annually.

Role of primary care in care of women who have had a diagnosis of GDM

Primary care needs to take on the responsibility for implementing all the above recommendations for women who have developed GDM, as most secondary care services no longer follow up people with GDM.

Summary

In relation to the six domains of core or essential competences of being a GP:

1 Primary care management

▷ An understanding of the possible adverse outcomes of pregnancy in
   women with diabetes.
▷ An understanding of the value of good blood glucose control at
   conception and early pregnancy in reducing the risk of congenital
   malformations.

2 Person-centred care

▷ Communication of the value of good blood glucose control in reducing
   adverse pregnancy outcomes to women with diabetes of childbearing
   age at every opportunity.

3 Specific problem-solving skills

▷ Understanding the need to stop diabetes medications that increase the
   risk of congenital malformations (mainly ACE inhibitors, AT2 agents
   and statins) when women with diabetes are contemplating pregnancy.
▷ Referring women with diabetes who say they are planning a pregnancy
   to a local, specific pre-pregnancy counselling programme.

4 A comprehensive approach

▷ Rapid referral of women with diabetes who become pregnant to a specialist diabetes/obstetric service as early in pregnancy as possible.

5 Community orientation

▷ Teaching the value of planning pregnancy and having good glucose control at conception to everyone with diabetes through local community diabetes support groups.

6 A holistic approach

▷ Ensuring that women with diabetes who are pregnant do not miss out on the antenatal preparation classes and other support that pregnant women without diabetes receive.

References

1 • Confidential Enquiry into Maternal and Child Health. *Diabetes and Pregnancy: are we providing the best care? Findings of a national enquiry. England, Wales and Northern Ireland* London: CEMACH, 2007.

2 • Temple R, Aldridge V, Greenwood R. Association between outcome of pregnancy and glycaemic control in pregnancy in type 1 diabetes: population based study *British Medical Journal* 2002; **325**: 1275–6.

3 • Kitzmiller J L, Gavin L A, Gin G D, *et al*. Preconception care of diabetes: glycaemic control prevents congenital abnormalities *Journal of the American Medical Association* 1991; **265**: 731–6.

4 • National Institute for Health and Clinical Excellence. *Clinical Guideline 63, Diabetes in Pregnancy: management of diabetes and its complications from pre-conception to the postnatal period* London: NICE, 2008, www.nice.org.uk/nicemedia/pdf/CG063NICEGuideline.pdf [accessed July 2009].

5 • Crowther C A, Hillier J E, Moss J R, *et al*. Australian Carbohydrate Intolerance Study in Pregnant Women (ACHIOS) Trial Group: effect of treatment of gestational diabetes mellitus on pregnancy outcomes *New England Journal of Medicine* 2005; **352**: 2477–86.

Thyroid disorders 10

Scenario 1

Frances is a 63-year-old woman who is an infrequent attendee at the practice. She has no significant previous medical history and is on no medications. She has made an appointment because she has been feeling increasingly tired and thinks she has slowed down over the past few months. She thinks she has put on around a stone in weight in the past 6 months. You elicit no other symptoms and physical examination is normal.

What investigations should be done?

▶ *Anaemia, Type 2 diabetes and hypothyroidism are all possible diagnoses to consider, so a full blood count, thyroid function tests and fasting glucose should be ordered.*

▶ *Her blood tests are all normal apart from her thyroid function tests, which reveal a low thyroxine (T4) level and raised thyroid-stimulating hormone (TSH) level.*

Hypothyroidism

The thyroid gland makes two hormones, T4 and tri-iodothyronine (T3). T4 itself is inactive and is converted in the body into T3, which is the active hormone that regulates cellular metabolism. When there is too little thyroid hormone available (hypothyroidism) the metabolism of the body slows down and significant symptoms may occur.

Symptoms of hypothyroidism

They may include:

▷ tiredness
▷ fatigue
▷ lethargy
▷ sensitivity to the cold

▷ dry skin and hair
▷ impaired concentration and memory
▷ increased weight with normal or reduced appetite
▷ constipation.

Patients may also complain of a change in their voice with increased hoarseness. Tingling in the hands may occur because carpal tunnel syndrome is quite common in hypothyroidism. Women may get heavier periods. If it occurs in childhood developmental delay may occur. Older people may develop problems with memory, impaired thinking and depression. If hypothyroidism is left untreated it can result in coma and even death.

Physical signs of hypothyroidism

These include: slow movements; bradycardia; cool, dry skin; thinning of the hair; slow tendon reflex relaxation time; and a hoarse voice. The face may take on a specific appearance termed 'myxoedema facies' in which it looks puffy due to the accumulation of subcutaneous fluid.

In some patients with hypothyroidism the thyroid gland may be enlarged, causing a 'goitre'. However, in others the thyroid is destroyed by the time of diagnosis and there is no goitre. Goitres were much commoner in the mid-nineteenth century and in people living in the centre of England. Having no proximity to the sea, the diet of this population did not contain fish, which is a source of iodine, required to produce the hormone thyroxine. Phrases such as 'Derbyshire neck' were used to describe these goitres.

In the UK, most people who develop hypothyroidism are diagnosed at a fairly early stage of the disease, and so may only have a few of the more non-specific symptoms listed above. None of the above symptoms and signs is sufficiently sensitive or specific for the diagnosis to be certain, so doctors need to have a strong index of suspicion and arrange the appropriate blood tests.

Diagnosing hypothyroidism

The typical blood test result shows a raised thyroid-stimulating hormone (TSH) level combined with a low T4 level.

Epidemiology of hypothyroidism

The prevalence in the UK of spontaneous hypothyroidism is thought to be around 2 per cent. It is 10 times more common in women than in men.[1] The raw prevalence data for hypothyroidism recorded in the Quality and

Outcomes Framework (QoF) in the UK for 2006/7 was 2.5 per cent.[2] This means a typical GP practice of 6000 patients will have around 140–50 patients with hypothyroidism.

Causes of hypothyroidism

There are two main causes in the UK that account for over 90 per cent of cases. These are, first, autoimmunity and, second, as a side effect of treatment of thyroid cancer or hyperthyroidism. In autoimmune thyroid disease the thyroid cells are destroyed by lymphocytes. It is accompanied by the presence of thyroid peroxidase (TPO) auto-antibodies in the blood, and so these are helpful in establishing the diagnosis.

There is an association between different autoimmune diseases. Someone with Type 1 diabetes has a higher prevalence of thyroid disease and coeliac disease compared with someone without Type 1 diabetes. Children with Type 1 diabetes should be screened for thyroid disease at diagnosis and 3-yearly thereafter.[3]

In people with hyperthyroidism or thyroid cancer, treatment often involves surgery or radioiodine treatment. These remove or destroy the diseased gland but often result in a significant proportion of patients developing hypothyroidism.

Treatment of hypothyroidism

Levothyroxine is the standard thyroid replacement therapy used in the UK. Treatment is usually started with a small dose and up-titrated until the symptoms of hypothyroidism are reversed and the blood TSH level is normalised.

A small dose (usually 25 mcg) is used initially, especially in older people, to minimise the risk of precipitating an adverse cardiac event.

Monitoring thyroid function in people taking levothyroxine

TSH monitoring is done on a regular basis to determine the correct dose of replacement therapy. The pituitary is very sensitive to changes in circulating levels of thyroid hormones and the amount of TSH secreted is a very clear indicator of the amount of thyroid hormones there are in circulation.

Measurement of serum T3 or T4 levels on their own are not recommended for monitoring thyroid hormone replacement in primary hypothyroidism. This is because the levels may change throughout the day after ingestion of the tablet and the levels do not reflect the tissue response to thyroid hormone in the way that TSH does. If, for example, a patient with hypothyroidism omits to take his or her levothyroxine for a few weeks the TSH levels will rise, but the T4 level will be normal if the patient remembers to take the levothyroxine the day before the blood test.

Thyroid function tests are usually checked annually in someone who is on a stable dose of thyroxine. This will enable the QoF criteria to be fulfilled.

Prescription exemption for levothyroxine

Hypothyroidism requiring treatment with levothyroxine replacement therapy qualifies a patient to obtain a prescription exemption certificate, which means that he or she does not have to pay for prescriptions of any medications available on the NHS. This certificate requires a countersignature from a doctor.

Subclinical hypothyroidism

Here the TSH levels are elevated but free thyroid hormone levels are within the normal range. This may be a precursor of clinical hypothyroidism, but there is still debate over whether it causes symptoms and should be treated. Treatment will therefore be a matter for individual clinical evaluation and discussion between patient and doctor. There is consensus that treatment with levothyroxine is usually worthwhile if repeated TSH levels exceed 10 iu/ml.[1]

Hypothyroidism in the Quality and Outcomes Framework

There are two clinical indicators for hypothyroidism in the QoF. These are:

▷ **thyroid 1** ▶ the practice can produce a register of patients with hypothyroidism (2 points)
▷ **thyroid 2** ▶ the percentage of patients with hypothyroidism with thyroid function tests recorded in the previous 15 months (6 points).

Scenario 1 revisited

Frances is started on levothyroxine 25 mcg and reviewed after 1 month. Although she felt less tired, her TSH remained elevated and so the dose was increased to 50 mcg. She was reviewed after another month with a repeat TSH, which was still elevated although Frances now felt well. The dose was increased to 75 mcg, and one further dose titration to 100 mcg was needed a month later before her TSH became normal. She has been maintained on this dose of 100 mcg and has checks on her TSH every 6 months.

Around 100 to 150 mcg of levothyroxine daily is the usual dose range to stabilise many adults with hypothyroidism.

Hyperthyroidism

Hyperthyroidism is caused by an excess circulation of free thyroxine (T4) and/or free triiodothyronine. There is an associated suppression of TSH.

Scenario 2

Bernadette is a 25-year-old woman who presents with a 2-month history of anxiety and palpitations. She has a 4-year-old child whom she looks after at home. She has no significant previous medical history. In discussion she says she has lost 5 kg in weight over this period. On examination she has a regular pulse rate of 108 beats per minute, a slight tremor of her outstretched hands, and you think there is a modest enlargement of her thyroid gland. Her eyes appear to be normal.

▶ *You order a series of blood tests including thyroid function. All are normal except the TSH, which is less than 0.1, and the T4 level is raised at 42.7 iu/ml.*

Symptoms of hyperthyroidism

These may include:

▷ anxiety and agitation
▷ palpitations
▷ weight loss despite a good appetite
▷ heat intolerance
▷ poor sleep
▷ sweating.

In some forms there are associated eye problems including exophthalmos, lid lag and proptosis.

Older patients may complain of heart problems, with a fast or irregular heartbeat, breathlessness and ankle swelling, whereas children tend to have a short attention span and hyperactivity.

Signs of hyperthyroidism

These may include:

▷ shake and/or a tremor
▷ hot hands
▷ a fast or irregular heartbeat
▷ inability to sit still
▷ flushing of the face and upper body
▷ brisk tendon reflexes
▷ an enlarged thyroid gland (goitre)
▷ prominent or bulging eyes (exophthalmos).

Many people today are diagnosed in the early stages of the condition because of increased awareness and early biochemical testing, so most people do not have all the 'classical' symptoms and signs mentioned. In the early stages the symptoms and signs are not very specific or sensitive, and so it is possible to go undiagnosed unless the diagnosis is considered and the appropriate blood tests arranged.

Diagnosing hyperthyroidism

The TSH is suppressed and the T4 and/or T3 levels are elevated.

Epidemiology of hyperthyroidism

The prevalence in women is around 0.5 per cent in the UK and it is about ten times more common in women than in men.[1] There are no clinical indicators for hyperthyroidism in the QoF, so no prevalence data is indicated.

Causes of hyperthyroidism

The two main causes in the UK, which account for over 90 per cent of cases, are autoimmunity causing stimulation of the thyroid gland and overproduction of thyroid hormones by benign tumours of the thyroid gland.

In autoimmune hyperthyroidism the thyroid cells are stimulated by an abnormal antibody that is specifically targeted at the TSH-receptor on the thyroid gland, causing stimulation of the thyroid to produce excess T4 and/or T3. The stimulation can cause the thyroid cells to grow and, together with an immune cell infiltration in the gland, can cause thyroid enlargement or goitre.

Autoimmune thyroid disease was described by an Irish doctor called Robert Graves and it is often called Graves's disease. It is accompanied by the presence of TSH-receptor antibodies in the blood and very frequently by thyroid peroxidase (TPO) auto-antibodies, which may both be useful in establishing the diagnosis.

About a third of people with Graves's disease develop thyroid eye disease or Graves's ophthalmolopothy. They can have symptoms of protruding eyes (exophthalmos), lid lag, sore and gritty eyes, and, more rarely, double vision and sight problems.

The other common cause of hyperthyroidism in the UK is from the development of one or more benign thyroid adenomas that secrete excess thyroid hormone in an unregulated manner. This condition of nodular hyperthyroidism is more common with advancing age. It is often called a solitary toxic nodule if there is only one, or a toxic multinodular goitre if there are several.

There are several rarer causes of hyperthyroidism, including several forms of thyroiditis, an inflammation of the thyroid gland. Hashimoto's thyroiditis typically affects women aged 55–75. It is an autoimmune disorder associated with positive thyroid antibodies. It commonly goes on to cause hypothyroidism, after an initial toxic phase. Subacute (de Quervain's) thyroiditis is characterised by pain in the gland and can present suddenly. Patients usually have a small, tender thyroid gland and a grossly elevated erythrocyte sedimentation rate (ESR). There is often a history of a preceding flu-like illness and a variety of viruses have been implicated in the condition including mumps, coxsackievirus and adenoviruses. Postpartum thyroiditis is usually transient and presents 3 to 6 months after delivery. The thyroid swelling is usually insignificant and the symptoms of thyrotoxicosis are mild.

All these forms of hyperthyroidism are termed 'primary' in that all result from an excessive release of hormones from the thyroid gland. Secondary hyperthyroidism occurs very rarely and is caused by a problem with overproduction of TSH from the pituitary gland. In this secondary hyperthyroidism there is a normal or raised TSH level.

Another cause of secondary hyperthyroidism is due to an excessive dose of levothyroxine taken to control hypothyroidism!

Subclinical hyperthyroidism

This is the term used to describe a condition of suppressed TSH but with normal T3 and T4 levels. Most endocrinologists regard this as a precursor of overt hyperthyroidism, but there is some debate as to whether it should be treated.[4] At present treatment is a matter for individual clinical evaluation and discussion between patient and doctor, although there is a consensus that treatment may be worthwhile in the elderly, particularly if the patient has atrial fibrillation or osteoporosis.[4]

111

Treatment of Graves's disease and nodular hyperthyroidism

ANTITHYROID DRUGS

Carbimazole at a usual dose of 40 mg per day or propylthiouracil at a dose of 300 mg per day reduce the production of thyroid hormones in most people with hyperthyroidism due to Graves's disease or nodular hyperthyroidism. In Graves's disease treatment is usually needed for between 6 months and 2 years. This results in long-term remission in about 50 per cent of people. The dose of drug can either be adjusted every 6 to 8 weeks according to the T4 level, to keep the T4 level in the normal range (this is called the titrated dose regime), or a fixed higher dose of antithyroid drug is given and levothyroxine replacement added to maintain a normal level of T4 (this is called the block and replace regime).

Side effects of the antithyroid drugs include a transient skin rash, muscle aches and very rarely agranulocytosis, which occurs in fewer than 0.2 per cent of patients and occurs usually within the first 3 months of therapy.[5] It usually reverses on stopping the drug.

It is important to warn patients on carbimazole therapy to see their doctor if they develop a persistent fever or sore throat. Persisting signs of infection mean that a full blood count will need to be arranged to exclude this rare complication of agranulocytosis.

BETA BLOCKERS

These do not cure the hyperthyroidism but do help to block some of its cardiac symptoms. Beta blockers may be usefully started at the same time as an antithyroid drug to enable people with hyperthyroidism to feel better until the antithyroid drug has time to work. They help to reduce tremor, palpitations and tachycardia. A dose of propranolol of 20–40 mg t.d.s. is often used where there are no contraindications to beta blockers.

RADIOIODINE TREATMENT

The radioactive isotope of iodine I-131 is taken up and concentrated selectively by the thyroid gland. There it gradually destroys the overactive thyroid tissue over a period of 6 weeks to 6 months after a single dose. Some hospital centres use a large dose to ablate the thyroid gland and then give levothyroxine replacement; other hospital centres use a smaller dose to preserve some thyroid function so that levothyroxine is not needed. Patients are monitored regularly for developing hypothyroidism and the need for levothyroxine replacement therapy. It is a safe treatment and there has been no overall excess of cancers after hundreds of thousands of patient years of follow-up.[6] There is no damage to future fertility but women are advised not to become pregnant for 6 months and men not to father a child for 4 months.

Surgical treatment for hyperthyroidism

Another approach is surgery to remove most or all the thyroid gland (sub-total or total thyroidectomy is another way of treating hyperthyroidism), which some patients may prefer. It is also the treatment of choice in people with very large thyroid swellings, people with allergy to antithyroid drugs, severe thyroid eye problems, and in severe hyperthyroidism in pregnancy. Prior to surgery, hyperthyroidism must be controlled with antithyroid drugs to make the anaesthetic safe. This is because an anaesthetic in a patient with uncontrolled hyperthyroidism has a high risk of precipitating a dangerous hyperthyroid crisis called a 'thyroid storm'.

Recurrent laryngeal nerve palsy can occur through damage to the nerve at operation and is said to occur in around 1 per cent of cases. Damage to the parathyroid glands can also occur, resulting in problems with low serum calcium levels. However, this is usually transient.

Treatment of thyroiditis

Many forms are self-limiting so that no antithyroid treatment is needed. Beta blockers may be helpful in controlling symptoms until the situation abates.

Scenario 2 revisited

In discussion with Bernadette you decide to start her on propranolol 20 mg t.d.s. to help her symptoms and refer to an endocrinologist for further advice. The endocrinologist confirms the diagnosis of Graves's hyperthy-roidism with no eye involvement, and begins her on carbimazole therapy. After 2 months she feels well and her thyroid function tests are normal. The beta blocker is stopped and carbimazole therapy continued for a total of 12 months. However, 3 months after stopping she becomes hyperthyroid both clinically and biochemically again.

Carbimazole is restarted and after discussion with the endocrinologist she opts for radioiodine therapy, which is successful but results in hypothy-roidism some 6 months after treatment. This is controlled on 100 mcg of levothyroxine.

Summary

In relation to the six domains of core or essential competences of being a GP:

1 Primary care management

▷ Recognition of the signs and symptoms of hyperthyroidism and hypothyroidism, and their management in primary care.
▷ To ensure that people with hyperthyroidism and hypothyroidism have the appropriate follow-up and annual review.

2 Person-centred care

▷ To understand the impact of hypothyroidism and hyperthyroidism on the individual and his or her concerns.

3 Specific problem-solving skills

▷ To be able to modify the dose of thyroxine appropriately in someone with hypothyroidism from thyroid function test results.

4 A comprehensive approach

▷ Ensuring that the practice has the necessary register of people with hypothyroidism to fulfil the QoF requirements and so facilitate recall and follow-up with annual thyroid function tests.

5 Community orientation

▷ Where possible to diagnose and treat thyroid disorders in primary care.
▷ Remembering that patients with hypothyroidism on medication are entitled to free prescriptions.
▷ To ensure that people with hyperthyroidism on carbimazole receive the necessary review and follow-up by arrangement with a consultant endocrinologist as appropriate.

6 A holistic approach

▷ To understand the impact that disorders of the thyroid can have on individuals and their lives.

References

1 • Vanderpump M P J, Tunbridge W M G, French J M, *et al*. The incidence of thyroid disorders in the community: a twenty-year follow-up of the Whickham Survey *Clinical Endocrinology* 1995; **43(1)**: 55–68.

2 • The Information Centre. QOF 2006/7 Data Tables, www.ic.nhs.uk/statistics-and-data-collections/supporting-information/audits-and-performance/the-quality-and-outcomes-framework/qof-2006/07/qof-2006-07-data-tables [accessed July 2009].

3 • National Institute for Clinical Excellence. *Clinical Guideline 15, Type 1 Diabetes: diagnosis and management of type 1 diabetes in children, young people and adults* London: NICE, 2004.

4 • Surks M I, Ortiz E, Daniels G H, *et al*. Subclinical thyroid disease: scientific review and guidelines for diagnosis and management *Journal of the American Medical Association* 2004; **291**: 228–38.

5 • Tajiri J, Noguchi S, Murakami T, *et al*. Antithyroid drug-induced agranulocytosis: the usefulness of routine white blood cell count monitoring *Archives of Internal Medicine* 1990; **150**: 621–4.

6 • Franklyn J A, Maisonneuve P, Sheppard M, *et al*. Cancer incidence and mortality after radioiodine treatment for hyperthyroidism: a population-based cohort study *Lancet* 1999; **353**: 2111–15.

Rare endocrine problems

Hypopituitarism

Hypopituitarism was first described clinically in 1914. It is the inability of the pituitary gland to provide sufficient hormones adapted to the needs of the person.[1] It may be due to the inability of the gland to produce hormones or an insufficient supply of hypothalamic-releasing hormones. It is usually chronic and lifelong, requiring hormone replacement, unless surgical or medical treatment of the primary cause can restore normal function.

The anterior pituitary produces adrenocorticotrophic hormone (ACTH), thyroid-stimulating hormone (TSH), luteinising hormone (LH), follicle-stimulating hormone (FSH), prolactin and growth hormone (GH). The posterior pituitary is a storage organ for the hypothalamic hormones, antidiuretic hormone (ADH) and oxytocin.

Epidemiology of hypopituitarism

One population-based study in a Spanish population gave a prevalence of 45.5 cases per 100,000.[2] The main causes were tumours (61 per cent).

In patients with traumatic brain injury and subarachnoid haemorrhage (SAH), 35 per cent and 48 per cent had some degree of hypopituitarism,[1] which sometimes might go unrecognised. Thus an increased prevalence of hypopituitarism needs to be assumed.

There are no Quality and Outcomes Framework (QoF) points for this problem.

Causes of hypopituitarism

The main causes are brain damage, pituitary tumours, non-pituitary tumours, infections, infarction, and others (which include unknown causes labelled as idiopathic).

Signs and symptoms

Sometimes it is the signs and symptoms of the underlying disease causing the hypopituitarism that are obvious first. Tumours of the pituitary cause slowly progressive visual disturbances, classically a bitemporal hemianopia. Headaches may be an unspecific sign of a tumour.

Hypopituitarism itself may be subclinical and only come to light when suspected and when hormone levels are measured. However, its onset can sometimes be acute and severe, necessitating hospital admission for intensive care. Acute shortages of ACTH, TSH and ADH are potentially life threatening. Shortages of GH, FSH and LH in contrast cause chronic morbidity.

If hypopituitarism is suspected referral to an endocrinologist for further investigation is indicated.

The following table lists the clinical features and abnormalities seen with various hormone deficiencies arising from hypopituitarism.

Table 11.1 ○ *Clinical abnormalities in hormone deficiency*

ACTH	
▶ Chronic	Fatigue, pallor, weight loss, hypoglycaemia, hypotension
▶ Acute	Weakness, collapse, fever, shock, anaemia, hyponatraemia
TSH	Tiredness, cold intolerance, dry skin, weight gain, bradycardia, hypotension, hoarse voice
▶ Children	Development and growth retardation
GH	Decreased muscle mass and strength, visceral obesity, dyslipidaemia, premature atherosclerosis
▶ Children	Growth retardation
ADH	Polyuria and polydipsia, decreased urine osmolarity, hypernatraemia
FSH/LH	
Women	Infertility, oligomenorrhoea, osteoporosis, loss of libido
Men	Loss of libido, mood impairment, loss of body hair, decreased muscle mass, osteoporosis

Diagnosis of hypopituitarism

A combination of low peripheral and inappropriately low pituitary hormones indicates hypopituitarism. However, basal concentrations alone may not be conclusive owing to the pulsatile, circadian and situational secretion of some hormones.[1] Investigations therefore need to be undertaken in appropriate specialist centres.

Hormone replacement regimes

Once a diagnosis has been made, unless the underlying cause can be remedied, the person with hypopituitarism will need to take hormone replacement therapy for life. Adequate replacement therapy can greatly enhance the quality of life, morbidity and mortality associated with hypopituitarism.[1]

Table 11.2 ○ *Suitable replacement regimes*[1]

To replace ACTH	Oral dose of 10–25 mg hydrocortisone daily in divided doses
	Increase to 100–150 mg for surgery or infection
To replace TSH	Levothyroxine orally as needed
To replace ADH	Desmopressin orally 0.3–1.2 mg/daily
To replace GH	GH parenterally children 25–50 pg/kg/day
To replace LH/FSH	
▶ Women	Oral contraceptive pill
▶ Men	Testosterone gel or depot injection usually given every 3 months

Follow-up

People are usually reviewed every 6–12 months when stable. When patients with hypopituitarism get a severe infection, e.g. a chest infection, or if they have to be admitted for surgery, they need an increased dose of hydrocortisone as suggested above. Patients with hypopituitarism need to carry something (for example a MedicAlert bracelet) that will alert healthcare professionals to their condition and the need for replacement therapy should they be admitted unconscious, for example after a road traffic accident.

Adrenal disease – primary aldosteronism

Primary aldosteronism (or Conn's syndrome) was described by Dr J Conn over 50 years ago in a patient with an aldosterone-producing adenoma (APA) in the adrenal gland, which caused hypokalaemia and hypertension. At surgery a right adrenal gland tumour was removed that resulted in the almost total reversal of the metabolic abnormalities.[3] It is now thought that bilateral idiopathic hyperplasia of the adrenal glands make up around 60 per cent of cases, with APA making up 35 per cent. The remaining 5 per cent of cases are made up of another five rare subtypes.

Epidemiology

It was thought that primary aldosteronism was a rare form of hypertension, but it is now being recognised as one of the most common causes of secondary hypertension. It makes up 5–13 per cent of all patients with hypertension.[3]

When to consider the possibility of primary aldosteronism

In patients with:

▷ hypertension and hypokalaemia (regardless of presumed cause)
▷ treatment-resistant hypertension (three or more drugs and poor control)
▷ severe hypertension
▷ hypertension and an incidental adrenal mass
▷ hypertension at a young age.

How to screen

If suspected, referral to an endocrinologist is indicated. The specialist is likely to perform a screening test by measuring a morning (preferably between 08.00–10.00) ambulatory pared random plasma aldosterone concentration (PAC) and plasma renin activity (PRA). An increased PAC:PRA ratio is not diagnostic by itself, but should be followed by the demonstration of inappropriate aldosterone secretion. Aldosterone suppression testing can be performed with orally administered sodium chloride or with intravenous sodium chloride loading and measurement of PAC. Once diagnosed it is necessary to perform further investigations to discover which subtype it is.

Management

In patients with an APA or unilateral adrenal hyperplasia the operation of unilateral adrenalectomy results in normalisation of serum potassium in all, improvement of hypertension in all and cure of hypertension in between 30–60 per cent.[3]

In bilateral adrenal forms of the condition unilateral or bilateral adrenalectomy seldom corrects the hypertension so the treatment of choice is a mineralocorticoid receptor antagonist.[3]

Adrenal disease – Addison's disease

Adrenal insufficiency was first described by Addison in 1855 and has been called Addison's disease ever since.[4] In the last century the principle cause was tuberculosis but now autoimmune disease accounts for most of the cases presenting outside the newborn period.[4] Adrenal insufficiency occurs when at least 90 per cent of the adrenal cortex has been destroyed. As a result of this destruction not enough cortisol and not enough aldosterone is produced.

Epidemiology

Addison's disease is quite rare and affects around 120 people per million.

Symptoms and signs

It often presents with ill-defined fatigue and weakness. It can mimic a gastro-intestinal disorder or a psychiatric disease, especially depression. Adrenal insufficiency may cause persistent vomiting, anorexia, hypoglycaemia, and poor weight gain in a child.

It can cause unexplained weight loss, malaise, fatigue, muscular weakness, hyperkalaemia, hypotension, hypoglycaemia and generalised hyperpigmentation. This 'muddy' hyperpigmentation is due to elevation of melanocyte-stimulating hormone (MSH) and ACTH caused by compensatory activation of the hypothalamic-pituitary axis.

Diagnosing Addison's disease

In the early stages it can be very difficult to diagnose. A survey of patients who are members of the National Adrenal Diseases Foundation showed that 60 per cent had sought medical attention from two or more physicians before the correct diagnosis was even considered.

The most specific diagnostic test is the ACTH stimulation test. Cortisol levels are measured before and after a synthetic form of ACTH is given by injection. In the so-called short or rapid test cortisol is measured 30–60 minutes after the ACTH is given. The normal response is a rise in cortisol but in patients with adrenal insufficiency the response is poor or absent.

Management of Addison's disease

This involves replacing the hormones that the adrenal gland is failing to make. Cortisol is replaced by oral hydrocortisone tablets 10 to 25 mg daily in divided doses. Aldosterone is replaced by oral fludrocortisone tablets 0.05–0.2 mg once daily.

Endogenous adrenal secretion is increased in normal people in illness and during operations. Patients with Addison's disease therefore need their routine hydrocortisone dose to be tripled and given as three divided daily doses when they get a significant febrile illness. If a patient cannot tolerate oral tablets IM or IV hydrocortisone will need to be given.

Patients with Addison's disease should wear a MedicAlert bracelet or necklace and carry the accompanying emergency medical information card at all times. For major surgery administration of hydrocortisone IV will be needed peri- and post-operatively before tapering over several days to a maintenance dose. It is unnecessary to give mineralocorticoid replacement as long as the patient begins the operative period in adequate salt balance.[4]

Cushing's syndrome

Endogenous Cushing's syndrome is a condition resulting from prolonged inappropriate exposure to excessive cortisol secretion with the subsequent loss of the normal feedback mechanism of the hypothalamic-pituitary-adrenal axis and the normal circadian rhythm of cortisol secretion. It is quite rare.

Secondary (or iatrogenic) Cushing's syndrome is far more common and is related to use of glucocorticoid treatment.

Epidemiology of primary Cushing's syndrome

It is a relatively rare disorder with an estimated incidence of 5–6 cases per 1 million population.[4]

Causes of primary Cushing's syndrome

In most large series of patients with endogenous Cushing's syndrome 80 per cent are ACTH dependent secondary to a tumour hypersecreting ACTH; 80 per cent of these are pituitary adenomas. The other 20 per cent are ACTH independent.[5]

If endogenous Cushing's syndrome is suspected referral to an endocrinologist is indicated for investigation and management.

Features of Cushing's syndrome

It is a disorder in which excessive glucocorticoid levels cause alterations in many of the body's organ systems, in proportion to the length of time of exposure and magnitude of the raised glucocorticoid levels.

The most common symptoms are non-specific and consist of weight gain with redistribution of adipose mass centrally to face, trunk, neck and abdomen. There can be thinning of the skin with easy bruising, abdominal striae, poor wound healing, immune suppression causing opportunistic and fungal infections, rib fractures, hirsutism in women, acne and proximal muscle weakness. Children with Cushing's syndrome have decreased growth velocity. Depression is common, and in severe cases psychosis and suicide can occur.[6] Associated problems such as diabetes mellitus, hypertension and osteoporosis may occur.

Diagnosing Cushing's syndrome

Investigation is initially by discovering raised glucocorticoid levels and then carrying out further investigations to find the precise cause.

Normal serum cortisol levels show a circadian rhythm reaching a peak between 07.00–09.00 and then falling during the rest of the day. Patients with Cushing's syndrome either show complete abolition of this circadian rhythm or have a circadian rhythm but set at a much higher level. The best test is therefore to do a sleeping midnight cortisol measurement, but this requires hospital admission. Other studies have suggested that a late-night salivary cortisol level may be a sensitive way of detecting the condition.[5]

A dexamethasone suppression test and other complex endocrine testing may also be needed as part of the investigations.

Treatment of Cushing's syndrome

If the cause is found to be a pituitary adenoma hypersecreting ACTH, pituitary surgery can be performed. Recurrence rates after such microsurgery have been reported as being between 42–86 per cent.[6] Pituitary radiation can be considered if surgery fails.

Bilateral adrenalectomy is another option if pituitary surgery fails. With comprehensive educational efforts and careful clinical monitoring, life-long adrenal insufficiency requiring glucocorticoid and mineralocorticoid replacement can be safely managed with minimal morbidity.[6]

Iatrogenic Cushing's syndrome

Endogenous Cushing's syndrome is rare and many GPs will not have any patients with the condition on their practice register. However, the early signs of Cushing's syndrome, especially the 'moon face' appearance, will quite commonly be seen in patients on long-term steroid therapy, especially where moderate to high doses are required for several months. Such 'iatrogenic' Cushing's syndrome may occur in patients on long-term oral steroid therapy because of temporal arteritis, polymyalgia rheumatica, severe asthma, systemic lupus, severe rheumatoid arthritis and other chronic inflammatory conditions. There have also been case reports of iatrogenic Cushing's syndrome after regular and long-term use of high-potency steroid creams.[7] It has also been reported in patients with AIDS treated by ritonavir (a potent inhibitor of cytochrome P450) who are taking inhaled steroids.[8]

This form of Cushing's syndrome reverses once the steroid treatment is stopped.

Summary

In relation to the six domains of core or essential competences of being a GP:

1 Primary care management

▷ To have an awareness of these rare endocrine problems.
▷ To work with a specialist endocrinologist to agree the appropriate care and follow-up of anyone in the practice with one of these rare endocrine problems.

2 Person-centred care

▷ To understand the impact of one of these rare endocrine conditions on the individual.

3 Specific problem-solving skills

▷ To understand the need for increasing replacement therapy at times of illness and operations, and to support patients to increase therapy.

4 A comprehensive approach

▷ To understand the impact of rare endocrine disease on the individual.

5 Community orientation

▷ To ensure that the patient receives appropriate follow-up for his or her rare endocrine condition.

6 A holistic approach

▷ To consider the psycho-social impact of conditions little known about by the general public.

References

1 • Schneider H J, Aimaretti G, Kreitschmann-Andermahr I, *et al*. Hypopituitarism *Lancet* 2007; **369**: 1461–70.

2 • Regal M, Paramo C, Sierra S M, *et al*. Prevalence and incidence of hypopituitarism in an adult Caucasian population in northwestern Spain *Clinical Endocrinology* 2001; **55**: 735–40.

3 • Young W F. Primary aldosteronism: renaissance of a syndrome *Clinical Endocrinology* 2007; **66**: 607–18.

4 • Ten S, New M, MacLaren N. Addison's disease *Journal of Clinical Endocrinology and Metabolism* 2001; **86**: 2909–22.

5 • Makras P, Toloumis G, Papadogias D, *et al*. The diagnosis and differential diagnosis of endogenous Cushing's syndrome *Hormones* 2006; **5**: 231–50.

6 • Findling J W, Raff H. Cushing's syndrome: important issues in diagnosis and management *Journal of Clinical Endocrinology and Metabolism* 2006; **91**: 3746–53.

7 • Gen R, Akbay E, Sezer K. Cushing's syndrome caused by topical steroid: a case report *American Journal of the Medical Sciences* 2007; **333**: 173–4.

8 • Samaras K, Pett S, Gowers A, *et al*. Iatrogenic Cushing's syndrome with osteoporosis and secondary adrenal failure in human immunodeficiency virus-infected patients receiving inhaled corticosteroids and ritonavir-boosted protease inhibitors: six cases *Journal of Clinical Endocrinology and Metabolism* 2005; **90**: 4394–8.

Index

127